T0264284

Vaccines and Immunology

Editors

AMY E.S. STONE
PHILIP H. KASS

VETERINARY CLINICS OF NORTH AMERICA: SMALL ANIMAL PRACTICE

www.vetsmall.theclinics.com

March 2018 • Volume 48 • Number 2

ELSEVIER

1600 John F. Kennedy Boulevard • Suite 1800 • Philadelphia, Pennsylvania, 19103-2899
http://www.vetsmall.theclinics.com

**VETERINARY CLINICS OF NORTH AMERICA: SMALL ANIMAL PRACTICE Volume 48, Number 2
March 2018 ISSN 0195-5616, ISBN-13: 978-0-323-58180-6**

Editor: Colleen Dietzler
Developmental Editor: Meredith Madeira

Veterinary Clinics of North America: Small Animal Practice (ISSN 0195-5616) is published bimonthly by Elsevier Inc., 360
Park Avenue South, New York, NY 10010-1710. Months of issue are January, March, May, July, September, and
November. Business and Editorial Offices: 1600 John F. Kennedy Blvd., Ste. 1800, Philadelphia, PA 19103-2899.
Customer Service Office: 3251 Riverport Lane, Maryland Heights, MO 63043. Periodicals postage paid at New York,
NY and additional mailing offices. Subscription prices are $325.00 per year (domestic individuals), $622.00 per year
(domestic institutions), $100.00 per year (domestic students/residents), $430.00 per year (Canadian individuals),
$773.00 per year (Canadian institutions), $469.00 per year (international individuals), $773.00 per year (international
institutions), and $220.00 per year (international and Canadian students/residents). To receive student/resident rate,
orders must be accompanied by name of affiliated institution, date of term, and the *signature* of program/residency
coordinator on institution letterhead. Orders will be billed at individual rate until proof of status is received. Foreign air
speed delivery is included in all *Clinics* subscription prices. All prices are subject to change without notice. **POSTMAS-
TER:** Send address changes to *Veterinary Clinics of North America: Small Animal Practice*, Elsevier Health Sciences
Division, Subscription Customer Service, 3251 Riverport Lane, Maryland Heights, MO 63043. Customer Service
(orders, claims, online, change of address): Elsevier Periodicals Customer Service, Elsevier Health Sciences Division
Subscription **Customer Service 3251 Riverport Lane Maryland Heights, MO 63043. Tel: 1-800-654-2452 (U.S.
and Canada); 314-447-8871 (outside U.S. and Canada). Fax: 314-447-8029. E-mail: journalscustomerservice-
usa@elsevier.com (for print support); journalsonlinesupport-usa@elsevier.com (for online support).**

Reprints. For copies of 100 or more of articles in this publication, please contact the Commercial Reprints Department,
Elsevier Inc., 360 Park Avenue South, New York, NY 10010-1710. Tel.: 212-633-3874; Fax: 212-633-3820; E-mail:
reprints@elsevier.com.

Veterinary Clinics of North America: Small Animal Practice is also published in Japanese by Inter Zoo Publishing
Co., Ltd., Aoyama Crystal-Bldg 5F, 3-5-12 Kitaaoyama, Minato-ku, Tokyo 107-0061, Japan.

Veterinary Clinics of North America: Small Animal Practice is covered in *Current Contents/Agriculture, Biology and Environmental Sciences, Science Citation Index, ASCA, MEDLINE/PubMed (Index Medicus), Excerpta Medica,* and *BIOSIS.*

Contributors

EDITORS

AMY E.S. STONE, BS, DVM, PhD
Clinical Assistant Professor, Service Chief of Primary Care and Dentistry, Small Animal Clinical Sciences, Gainesville, Florida, USA

PHILIP H. KASS, DVM, MPVM, MS, PhD
Diplomate, American College of Veterinary Preventive Medicine (Specialty in Epidemiology); Vice Provost for Academic Affairs, Professor of Analytic Epidemiology, Department of Population Health and Reproduction, School of Veterinary Medicine, Department of Public Health Sciences, School of Medicine, University of California, Davis, Davis, California, USA

AUTHORS

PHILIP J. BERGMAN, DVM, MS, PhD
Diplomate, American College of Veterinary Internal Medicine (Oncology); Director, Clinical Studies, VCA, Los Angeles, California, USA; Oncologist, Katonah-Bedford Veterinary Center, Bedford Hills, New York, USA; Adjunct Associate Member, Memorial Sloan-Kettering Cancer Center, New York, New York, USA

JOHN A. ELLLIS, DVM, PhD
Diplomate, American College of Veterinary Pathologists; Diplomate, American College of Veterinary Microbiologists; Professor, Department of Veterinary Microbiology, Western College of Veterinary Medicine, University of Saskatchewan, Saskatoon, Saskatchewan, Canada

MICHAEL JAMES FRANCIS, PhD, EurProBiol, CBiol, FRSB, HonAssocRCVS
Managing Director, BioVacc Consulting Ltd, Amersham, Buckinghamshire, United Kingdom

LAUREL J. GERSHWIN, DVM, PhD
Diplomate, American College of Veterinary Microbiology; Distinguished Professor of Immunology, Department of Pathology, Microbiology and Immunology, School of Veterinary Medicine, University of California, Davis, Davis, California, USA

SYDNEY W. JONES, BS
Veterinary Research Student, College of Veterinary Medicine, Texas A&M University, College Station, Texas, USA

PHILIP H. KASS, DVM, MPVM, MS, PhD
Diplomate, American College of Veterinary Preventive Medicine (Specialty in Epidemiology); Vice Provost for Academic Affairs, Professor of Analytic Epidemiology, Department of Population Health and Reproduction, School of Veterinary Medicine, Department of Public Health Sciences, School of Medicine, University of California, Davis, Davis, California, USA

RICHARD A. SQUIRES, BVSc, PhD
Associate Professor, Companion Animal Medicine, Section Leader, Veterinary Clinical Sciences, Discipline, Veterinary Science, James Cook University, Townsville, Queensland, Australia

IAN R. TIZARD, BVMS, PhD, DSc, ACVM
University Distinguished Professor of Immunology, Department of Veterinary Pathobiology, College of Veterinary Medicine, Texas A&M University, College Station, Texas, USA

Contents

Recent Advances in Vaccine Technologies   231

Michael James Francis

> This article discusses some recent advances in vaccine technologies with particular reference to their application within veterinary medicine. It highlights some of the key inactivated/killed approaches to vaccination, including natural split-product and subunit vaccines, recombinant subunit and protein vaccines, and peptide vaccines. It also covers live/attenuated vaccine strategies, including modified live marker/differentiating infected from vaccinated animals vaccines, live vector vaccines, and nucleic acid vaccines.

Another Look at the "Dismal Science" and Jenner's Experiment   243

John A. Elllis

> The follow-up to Jenner's experiment, routine vaccination, has reduced more disease and saved more vertebrate lives than any other iatrogenic procedure by orders of magnitude. The unassailability of that potentially provocative cliché has been ciphered in human medicine, even if it is more difficult in our profession. Most public relations headaches concerning vaccines are a failure to communicate, often resulting in overly great expectations. Even in the throes of a tight appointment schedule remembering and synopsizing (for clients), some details of the dismal science can make practice great again.

Veterinary Oncology Immunotherapies   257

Philip J. Bergman

> The ideal cancer immunotherapy agent should be able to discriminate between cancer and normal cells, be potent enough to kill small or large numbers of tumor cells, and be able to prevent recurrence of the tumor. Tumor immunology and immunotherapy are among the most exciting and rapidly expanding fields; cancer immunotherapy is now recognized as a pillar of treatment alongside traditional modalities. This article highlights approaches that seem to hold particular promise in human clinical trials and many that have been tested in veterinary medicine.

Adverse Reactions to Vaccination: From Anaphylaxis to Autoimmunity   279

Laurel J. Gershwin

> Vaccines are important for providing protection from infectious diseases. Vaccination initiates a process that stimulates development of a robust

and long-lived immune response to the disease agents in the vaccine. Side effects are sometimes associated with vaccination. These vary from development of acute hypersensitivity responses to vaccine components to local tissue reactions that are annoying but not significantly detrimental to the patient. The pathogenesis of these responses and the consequent clinical outcomes are discussed. Overstimulation of the immune response and the potential relationship to autoimmunity is evaluated in relation to genetic predisposition.

Dogs and cats entering animal shelters are at high risk of acquiring one or more contagious infectious diseases. Such animals may be severely stressed, exhausted, and unwell, as well as malnourished and parasitized. The typically high throughput of shelter animals, many of them young and of unknown vaccination status, plays a role. Vaccines are a crucially important part of the management approach to limiting morbidity, mortality, and spread of infection. Guidelines for the use of vaccines in shelters have been published and are reviewed and discussed in this article.

Recently published guidelines have made specific vaccine recommendations purported to potentially reduce the incidence of feline injection-site sarcomas (FISS). These recommendations have largely been based on experimental models of inflammation under different vaccine formulations. In none of these studies did sarcomas occur. It is scientifically untenable to address FISS risk based on propensity of vaccines to elicit differential inflammatory responses if none of those responses led to sarcoma development. Although the recommendations may ultimately be found to be prescient and valid, it will take considerable additional research before this can happen. Until then, such guidelines must be regarded with skepticism.

The complex commensal microbiota found on body surfaces controls immune responses and the development of allergic and inflammatory diseases. New genetic technologies permit investigators to determine the composition of the complex microbial populations found on these surfaces. Changes in the microbiota (dysbiosis) as a result of antibiotic use, diet, or other factors thus influence the development of many diseases in the dog and cat. The most important of these include chronic gastrointestinal disease; respiratory allergies, such as asthma; skin diseases, especially atopic dermatitis; and some autoimmune diseases.

There are many autoimmune diseases that are recognized in domestic animals. The descriptions of diseases provide examples of the magnitude of immune targets and the variable nature of autoimmune diseases. Other autoimmune diseases that are recognized in dogs, cats, and horses include immune-mediated thrombocytopenia, VKH (Vogt-Koyanagi-Harada) ocular disease (dogs), and Evans syndrome (which includes both immune-mediated anemia and immune-mediated thrombocytopenia).

VETERINARY CLINICS OF NORTH AMERICA: SMALL ANIMAL PRACTICE

Erratum

In the January 2018 issue (Volume 48, number 1), in the article on pages 31-43, "Feline Epilepsy," by Heidi Barnes Heller, the author's name was incorrectly written as Heidi Heller. The correct name for the author is Heidi Barnes Heller.

A corrected version of this article can be found online at http://vetsmall.theclinics.com/.

Vet Clin Small Anim 48 (2018) ix
https://doi.org/10.1016/j.cvsm.2017.12.013
0195-5616/18

Preface

Vaccinology and Immunology: Current Knowledge, New Discoveries, and Future Directions

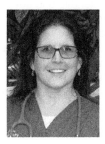 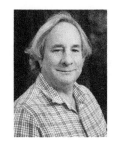

Amy E.S. Stone, BS, DVM, PhD   Philip H. Kass, DVM, MPVM, MS, PhD
Editors

Although the way ahead (for Immunology) is full of pitfalls and difficulties, this is indeed an exhilarating prospect. There is no danger of a shortage of forthcoming excitement in the subject. Yet, as always, the highlights of tomorrow are the unpredictabilities of today.
—César Milstein, PhD from Nobel Lecture (8 Dec 1984), collected in Tore Frängsmyr and Jan Lindsten (editors.), Nobel Lectures in Physiology or Medicine: 1981-1990 (1993), 267.

Immunology is a comparatively young scientific field that seems to advance with exhausting speed and complexity. It is also a fundamental discipline in veterinary medical science and clinical veterinary medicine. The pace with which it inexorably evolves and the explosion of the growth in the scientific literature can make it difficult for the academician studying these new discoveries, veterinary specialists translating research into practice, and certainly for the general practitioner to keep current with the latest information and pertinent findings. It is enigmatic, if not disheartening, that even in the face of the astonishing success of vaccination in controlling infectious diseases and saving lives throughout the world that there still appears to be residual public skepticism about the science and scientists underlying it. And yet its conjoining with pharmacotherapeutics represents medicine's greatest hope for the emergence of a new armament of chemical and biological weapons to fight infectious and even noninfectious disease.

As editors, we began contemplating this issue of *Veterinary Clinics of North America: Small Animal Practice* by wanting to cover topics about vaccinology and immunology that colleagues across our profession want and need to know more about. We want to

Vet Clin Small Anim 48 (2018) xi–xii
https://doi.org/10.1016/j.cvsm.2017.12.001
0195-5616/18/© 2017 Published by Elsevier Inc.   **vetsmall.theclinics.com**

challenge the reader to think beyond vaccination as a tool to prevent infectious disease in small animal general practice. We want veterinarians to understand the spectrum of research underlying vaccination recommendations and protocols. In addition, we hope to provide information that will give veterinarians a fundamental understanding of how vaccines work the way that they do as well as new directions for vaccine technologies.

In our attempt to meet our above wants and goals, we have compiled a unique selection of original, carefully reviewed articles in this issue of *The Veterinary Clinics of North America: Small Animal Practice.* We certainly visit concepts and controversies about vaccination technology and vaccination response (both intended and adverse); however, we also managed to encompass articles about oncologic immunotherapies, vaccination in group/shelter settings, microbiota's regulation of immunity, and newly emerging autoimmune diseases. While we did not manage to cover all of the topics we initially sought to, we certainly covered an impressive array.

We would like to thank our talented authors for their time and efforts to keep our understanding of veterinary immunology and vaccinology current and accurate. Each of them brought unique and provocative perspectives and critical thinking to this issue and to these concepts. It has been a privilege for us to edit this distinctive issue.

Amy E.S. Stone, BS, DVM, PhD
Small Animal Clinical Sciences
PO Box 100116
Gainesville, FL 32610, USA

Philip H. Kass, DVM, MPVM, MS, PhD
Department of Population Health and Reproduction
School of Veterinary Medicine
Department of Public Health Sciences
School of Medicine
University of California, Davis
1089 Veterinary Medicine Drive
Davis, CA 95616, USA

E-mail addresses:
stonea@ufl.edu (A.E.S. Stone)
phkass@ucdavis.edu (P.H. Kass)

Recent Advances in Vaccine Technologies

Michael James Francis, PhD, EurProBiol, CBiol, FRSB, HonAssocRCVS

KEYWORDS

- Vaccines • Inactivated • Attenuated • Subunit • Peptide • Vector • DIVA
- Nucleic acid

KEY POINTS

- Traditional vaccine technologies are based on killed/inactivated and live/attenuated approaches.
- Novel killed/inactivated vaccination strategies include antigen subunit, protein, and peptide vaccines.
- Novel live/attenuated vaccination strategies include modified live, marker/differentiating infected from vaccinated animals, vector, and nucleic acid vaccines.
- New vaccine technologies often find their first commercial application within veterinary medicine.

INTRODUCTION

Most vaccines that are available today rely on either inactivated (killed) or live attenuated (weakened) technologies. Such approaches have been successfully used to address many of the important veterinary and human diseases. However, both techniques have their limitations and associated potential problems.

Inactivated vaccines must be totally innocuous and noninfective. Problems with field outbreaks in the past have occasionally been attributed to incomplete inactivation. Such problems should not, and would not, exist if more reliable inactivants, inactivation procedures, and innocuity testing were used within the manufacturing process. Furthermore, because the manufacture of such vaccines involves the culture of large amounts of the infectious agent, there is a potential hazard to the personnel involved and the environment. Vaccines grown in eggs, tissue culture, or simply culture medium may contain unwanted "foreign" proteins, which could affect immunogenicity or be potentially allergenic/reactogenic. Finally, inactivated vaccines have certain limitations on their mode of presentation and as a consequence the nature of the immune response they can elicit. The response to vaccination may be limited

The author has nothing to disclose.
BioVacc Consulting Ltd, The Red House, 10 Market Square, Amersham, Buckinghamshire HP7 0DQ, UK
E-mail address: mike.francis@biovacc.com

Vet Clin Small Anim 48 (2018) 231–241
https://doi.org/10.1016/j.cvsm.2017.10.002
0195-5616/18/© 2017 Elsevier Inc. All rights reserved.

and of short duration with adjuvants or immunostimulants required to enhance their overall immunogenicity/efficacy.

Attenuated vaccines must be precisely controlled and characterized in order to provide the required level of protective immunity without causing significant disease symptoms within the host animal. There is also a low risk that the attenuated antigen may revert to full virulence, and careful reversion to virulence safety studies must be carried out. Furthermore, in culturing the vaccine antigen, it is possible that other infectious agents may be introduced that could themselves lead to undesired side effects when the vaccine is used in the field.

Because of these and other reasons, including protective efficacy, economy of manufacture, and whether the infectious agent can be produced in vitro, scientists have turned their attention more and more to the new vaccine technologies. These vaccine technologies include split-product, subunit, isolated protein, peptide, marker vaccine, live vector, and nucleic acid approaches.

KILLED VACCINE STRATEGIES
Natural Split-Product and Subunit Vaccines

By identifying suitable subunit, protein, or peptide antigens as vaccine candidates, natural split-product and subunit vaccines must be delivered to the target animals in order to elicit the desired protective immune response. The simplest and most basic form of subunit vaccine is one in which the infectious agent has simply been disassembled or broken up into its component parts. Some current influenza vaccines, known as split-product vaccines, consist of formalin inactivated virus that has been treated in order to lyse the viral envelope and release both the external envelope proteins and the internal nuclear and matrix proteins. A further refinement has been to use the purified envelope glycoproteins hemagglutinin and neuraminidase alone in a subunit vaccine in order to reduce the risk of any toxic side effects. Unfortunately, split-product and subunit vaccines for influenza have tended to have reduced immunogenicity when compared with whole virus products. Attempts to improve this situation have concentrated on modifying antigen presentation by delivering the viral glycoproteins within lipid vesicles, which can be composed of either virus-derived lipids (virosomes) or added nonviral lipids (liposomes).[1] In this way, artificial "empty" viruses can be created that can display improved immunogenicity. Polymeric preparations of isolated proteins in the form of micelles are also more immunogenic than the protein monomer.[2] In recent times, such multimeric presentation systems are often collectively referred to as virus-like particles or VLPs.[3] A development that offers both polymeric presentation and built-in adjuvant activity, for further enhancing immunogenicity, is the immunostimulating complex or ISCOM.[4] The first successful commercial veterinary application of this technology was for equine influenza,[5] and these vaccines have been studied for mucosal delivery.[6] Split product and cell culture subunit vaccines are also currently marketed for feline leukemia virus (FeLV) disease. Although each has been shown to be immunogenic, their overall degree of efficacy particularly in the face of an oronasal challenge has been inconsistent. However, once again by presenting the surface glycoprotein gp70/85 of FeLV in an ISCOM, neutralizing antibodies were elicited in all vaccinated cats, and complete protection was demonstrated against a subsequent oronasal challenge.[7]

As well as these new generations of veterinary viral subunit vaccines, many current bacterial vaccines are based on toxin or pilus subunits. Although antitoxin antibodies will neutralize the harmful effects of the bacterial infection, antipilus antibodies will block colonization by preventing attachment. Good examples are the F4 (K88),

F5 (K99), F6 (987P), F7 (F41), and F18 fimbrial adhesion antigens of enterotoxigenic *Escherichia coli* (ETEC), which in current vaccines are used to prevent neonatal diarrhea in calves and pigs. Indeed *E coli* strains engineered to overproduce these antigens were probably the first examples of the use of recombinant DNA technology to develop improved commercial vaccines.[8]

Recombinant Subunit and Protein Vaccines

Vaccines produced using overexpressed proteins recovered from genetically modified *E coli* provide a link between natural subunit vaccines and those derived using recombinant DNA technology. Although subunit vaccines produced from the natural infectious agent still fulfill an important role, the cost of producing and purifying immunogen can be prohibitive. Indeed, once the immunogenic proteins have been identified, it becomes the goal of many researchers to produce large quantities of those proteins in a sufficiently pure form to generate safe and effective vaccines. The emergence of recombinant DNA technology meant that foreign genes could be inserted into expression vectors and then introduced into cells that act as "production factories" for the foreign proteins encoded for by those genes. In many cases, this provides a relatively inexhaustible and cheap source of protein from the infectious agent for vaccination studies.

1. Bacterial expression: The first recombinant expression systems were established using *E coli* bacteria. This was the natural choice because it had been used to develop the early concepts and understanding of molecular biology. This expression system can provide relatively large quantities of defined proteins and was thus heralded as the answer for many subunit vaccines. However, because of the fact that prokaryotic cells have different mechanisms for processing and trafficking, expressed proteins are often incorrectly folded. In addition, signal sequences, glycosylation sites, and disulfide bonds, which occur in many candidate vaccine proteins, can either result in toxicity, insolubility, or rapid degradation within the bacterium. Nevertheless, one of the first recombinant veterinary vaccines to be successfully produced was based on the gp70 surface glycoprotein of FeLV expressed in *E coli*, known as the p45 protein.[9]

2. Yeast expression: The widespread use of *Saccharomyces cerevisiae*, baker's yeast, as an industrial microorganism has made it a natural choice for an alternative antigenic protein expression system. It has the added advantage, over prokaryotic systems, that posttranslational modification of proteins is carried out in a manner similar to that used by higher eukaryotic cells, and therefore, recombinant proteins are more likely to be correctly folded. Yeast-expressed proteins will also be glycosylated, although this glycosylation will be distinct from that carried out by mammalian cells. Further developments in yeast expression have concentrated on exploring the potential of another strain of yeast (*Pichia pastoris*), which has been used to express human hepatitis B vaccines based on the virus surface antigen (HBsAg) at levels as high as 400 mg/L. These expression levels are 10-fold higher than reported levels for this protein in *S cerevisiae*.[10]

3. Insect cell expression: A more recent and highly novel expression system has been developed using insect ovarian cells from *Spodoptera frugiperda* infected with a baculovirus vector, *Autographa californica* nuclear polyhedrosis virus. These viruses possess a strong promoter that controls the production of a 29-kDa polyhedron protein, which accumulates eventually to constitute up to 50% of total infected cell protein. Therefore, by replacing the polyhedrin gene with a selected foreign gene, high levels of recombinant protein may be produced. These proteins

will also undergo posttranslational modification, including glycosylation, phosphorylation, and signal peptide cleavage. However, once again the glycosylation pattern is known to be different from that seen on mammalian cell-derived proteins. Expression levels as high as 1 g per liter could be expected, although actual levels can vary considerably from 1 to 600 mg depending on the antigen. Insect cell expression has been successfully used in veterinary vaccines against porcine circovirus type 2[11] and classical swine fever (CSF).[12]

4. Mammalian cell expression: Because many veterinary pathogens will infect and replicate in cultured mammalian cells, they would appear to be the natural choice for an expression system if one desires authentically processed proteins for a subunit vaccine. However, they do present several technical problems, and expression levels can be somewhat lower that those achieved using the alternative expression systems described above. Nevertheless, several systems are available for the expression of proteins in mammalian cells and have been successfully used to express candidate vaccine proteins for bovine viral diarrhea (BVD),[13] CSF,[14] and VLPs for Japanese encephalitis virus.[15]

5. Plant cell expression: An additional emerging expression system that warrants mention is the use of plant cells. Although in the past plant geneticists have largely concentrated on crop improvement, some recent studies have shown that plants may provide a useful expression system for mammalian proteins. To express foreign genes in plants, it is necessary to splice a plant promoter, terminator, and, generally, a regulatory sequence onto cloned complementary DNA. Selectable markers may also be incorporated to facilitate identification of recombinants, and the expression hosts can be plant either cell cultures or whole plants. The first licensed vaccine to use this expression system was against Newcastle disease virus (NDV) infection in poultry,[16] and it is being investigated for many other vaccine applications, including infectious bronchitis virus, infectious bursal disease virus, ETEC, BVD, and bovine herpes virus.[17,18]

Peptide Vaccines

By identifying and sequencing important immunogenic sites on infectious agents, these can in many cases be mimicked using short chains of amino acid (peptides). The first indication that such peptides had vaccine potential was demonstrated in 1963 using a plant virus, tobacco mosaic virus. In this study, a chemically isolated hexapeptide fragment from the virus coat protein was coupled to bovine serum albumin and used to elicit rabbit antibodies that would neutralize the infectious virus. Two years later, a synthetic form of the same peptide was used to confirm this observation. However, it was more than 10 years before the next example of a peptide that elicited antivirus antibody appeared following work by Sela and colleagues on a virus that infects bacteria, MS2 bacteriophage.[19] The emergence of more accessible techniques for sequencing proteins in 1977, coupled with the ability readily to synthesize peptides developed by Merrifield in 1963,[20] led to an upsurge in experimental peptide vaccine research in the 1980s.[21] The first demonstration that peptides could elicit protective immunity in vivo in addition to neutralizing activity in vitro was obtained in 1982 using an animal virus, foot-and-mouth disease virus (FMDV).[22] A detailed study of both enzymically and chemically cleaved fragments of viral protein 1 (VP1) from the virus of FMDV serotype 0 had identified 2 regions between amino acids 138 to 154 and 200 to 213, which were found on the surface of the virus, and fragments containing these regions were able to induce neutralizing antibodies against the homologous virus. Studies using chemically synthesized peptides corresponding to several regions of VP1 led to the identification of similar sites on the molecule (141–160 and 200–213), which when coupled to a protein carrier, keyhole limpet hemocyanin (KLH), and inoculated into guinea pigs would raise neutralizing antibodies that could protect against experimental infection. Although in these early studies the peptide had an immunogenic activity that was only 1% or less of that seen with the inactivated virus particle on an equal weight basis, the levels of neutralizing antibody produced were several orders of magnitude greater than that obtained with the whole VP1 molecule. This observation in laboratory animal models has subsequently been supported by the demonstration of protective immunity to peptide vaccination in both cattle[23] and pigs.[24]

Once a candidate peptide is identified or predicted, then it must be delivered to the immune system in a suitable manner in order to elicit not just a high titer antipeptide response but also antipeptide antibodies that will recognize and neutralize the infectious agent. Indeed, there has been a widely held view that, due to their relatively small molecular size, peptides are poor immunogens and thus require carrier-coupling to enhance their immunogenicity. Because of this, there are many examples of elegantly defined peptides, which, having been coupled in an uncontrolled manner to large undefined carrier proteins, produced antipeptide antibodies that totally failed to recognize the native protein.

Defined peptides, which, having been coupled in an uncontrolled manner to large undefined carrier proteins, produced antipeptide antibodies that totally failed to recognize the native protein.[25] The concept that peptides behave like haptens is in many cases misguided. Experiments using the 141 to 160 peptide from FMDV have demonstrated that the role of KLH as a carrier in priming for a peptide response is fundamentally different from its role in hapten priming because an uncoupled peptide or peptide coupled to a different carrier (tetanus toxoid) could boost a response in peptide-KLH primed animals. This observation has led to the demonstration of helper T-cell and B-cell determinants on this relatively small peptide.[26] Indeed, it is now clear that uncoupled peptides can be immunogenic provided they contain appropriate antibody recognition sites (B-cell epitopes) as well as sites capable of eliciting T-cell help for antibody production (Th-cell epitopes). These Th-cell epitopes must interact with class II major histocompatibility complex (MHC) molecules on the surface of antigen-presenting cells and B cells and subsequently bind to a T-cell receptor in the form of a trimolecular complex. The Th cells will provide signals in the form of chemical messengers (lymphokines) to specific B cells, which result in differentiation, proliferation, and antibody production. With this knowledge, synthetic peptides can be constructed with appropriate sites for antibody production plus additional T-cell epitopes.[27,28] This approach has been further exploited using a peptide containing B-cell epitopes within a consensus sequence based on residues 129 to 169 of Asian type O viruses linked to a promiscuous artificial Th-cell site from measles virus, which has now been commercially licensed for use as an FMDV peptide vaccine in swine.[29]

The requirement for multiple copy peptide presentation has been investigated using recombinant DNA technology by fusing small peptide sequences to the genes coding for larger proteins in order to produce several novel constructs. The use of peptide sequences fused to bacterial proteins as immunogens has the potential advantage of a completely uniform and defined structure compared with the uncharacterized and variable nature of peptide/carrier conjugates prepared by chemical cross-linking. This approach has been used to express FMDV peptides fused to the N-terminus of B-galactosidase in E coli cells. B-galactosidase was chosen because it had been shown that antibodies can be produced to foreign proteins located at the N-terminus, and it was known to contain several helper T-cell sites. Preliminary experiments with B-galactosidase and TrpLE fusion proteins indicated that multiple copies of the inserted peptide sequence may be beneficial. Subsequently, the immunogenicity of 1, 2, or 4 copies of FMDV VP1 peptide 137 to 162 fused to the N-terminus of

B-galactosidase was studied in both laboratory animals and target species. The protein containing one copy of the viral determinant elicited only low levels of neutralizing antibody, whereas protective levels were elicited by proteins containing 2 or 4 copies of the determinant.[30] Furthermore, single inoculations of the 2-copy and 4-copy proteins containing as little as 2 μg or 0.8 μg of peptide, respectively, were sufficient to protect all laboratory animals against challenge infection. The equivalent of 40 μg of peptide in the 4-copy protein also protected pigs against challenge infection after one inoculation. Thus, the immunogenicity of the multiple copy peptide/B-galactosidase fusion proteins is similar to that obtained using a synthetic multiple antigen peptide system.[31]

A further development of the fusion protein concept for multiple peptide presentation has led to the production of particulate structures with epitopes repeated over their entire surface, similar to VLPs. The earliest examples of these are based on HBsAg, hepatitis B core antigen (HBcAg), and yeast Ty proteins, which spontaneously self-assemble into 22-, 27-, and 60-nm particles, respectively. It has been shown using HBcAg fusion particles (CFPs) that the immunogenicity of FMDV peptide can approach that of the inactivated virus. Indeed, as little as 0.2 μg of FMDV VP1 142 to 160 peptide corresponding to 10% of the fusion protein, presented on the surface of CFPs, gave full protection to guinea pigs.[32] In subsequent experiments, N-terminal CFPs were shown to be 100-fold more immunogenic than free disulfide dimer synthetic peptides containing B- and T-cell determinants and 10-fold more immunogenic than carrier-linked peptide. This activity appears to be dependent both on the provision of T-cell help from the HBcAg and on particle formation. CFPs are also immunogenic with or without conventional vaccine adjuvants in a wide range of species. Furthermore, systemic responses can be elicited by oral or nasal administration and in a T-cell–independent manner. This last property of the CFPs offers the possibility of developing vaccine-based therapies for immunocompromised individuals infected with immunodeficiency viruses.[33]

Although only a limited number of peptide-based vaccines have been licensed to date, they offer the opportunity of moving vaccines from relatively undefined biological entities to more defined pharmaceutical-like products, and they have now been used to elicit immune responses against a wide variety of veterinary viruses, including rabies virus, FeLV, bovine rotavirus, bovine enterovirus, canine parvovirus, respiratory syncytial virus, equine herpes virus, and bovine leukemia virus.[21]

LIVE VACCINE STRATEGIES
Modified Live Marker/Differentiating Infected from Vaccinated Animals Vaccines

New technology vaccines can also be used as a valuable tool in disease control and eradication programs by enabling the user to differentiate infected from vaccinated animals. These marker or DIVA (differentiating infected from vaccinated animals) vaccines can be recombinant deletion mutants of wild-type pathogens or subunit/peptide vaccines. They will require an accompanying diagnostic test for screening, and they can make it possible for vaccines to be used more readily in nonendemic situations. Early examples of such rationally attenuated glycoprotein deletion mutants have been used for the control of pseudorabies and CSF in pigs and infectious bovine rhinotracheitis in cattle.[34]

Live Vectored Vaccines

Live attenuated vaccines offer several distinct advantages over conventional inactivated and subunit vaccines. By replicating in the host, they more accurately mimic natural infection, and they are often easy to administer, provide long-lived immunity, and stimulate a more "comprehensive" immune response, including humoral antibodies, secretory antibodies, and cytotoxic T cells. For these reasons, scientists have investigated ways of delivering subunit or peptide vaccines using live vectors.

1. Virus vectors: Most virus vector studies have concentrated on relatively large DNA viruses, in particular, poxviruses, herpesviruses, and adenoviruses. The most common virus vector to be applied experimentally is the orthopoxvirus vaccinia, successfully used in the vaccination campaign to eradicate smallpox.[35] The observation that a 9000-base-pair segment of the vaccinia virus genome could be deleted without affecting either its infectivity or its ability to replicate led to the development of recombinant vaccinia viruses with inserted foreign genes. Indeed, it has been shown that up to 25,000 base pairs of foreign DNA can be inserted into the virus, which offers the potential for inserting several genes into a single vector to produce a multicomponent vaccine. Despite these numerous positive observations, there are several potential problems associated with the use of vaccinia. In producing the initial recombinant, it is possible that cell tropism and pathogenicity may be affected. Because of its broad host range, there may also be problems with virus dissemination and recombination with other poxviruses under field conditions. However, the biggest question is undoubtedly that of safety. Despite its excellent track record in the smallpox eradication campaign, vaccinia has been known on very rare occasions to cause serious adverse reactions. In spite of these reservations, vaccinia recombinants have been used under strict supervision in the field in an attempt to control the spread of rabies in wildlife in Europe and North America. In view of its promising properties, much attention has been given to further rational attenuation of the vaccinia virus. For example, insertion into the TK gene has been shown to produce a marked reduction in pathogenicity, and further deletions or insertions have been investigated to produce a safer vector for general vaccination purposes. One such vector is known as modified vaccinia virus Ankora, and this has been recently used to develop a vaccine against Middle East respiratory syndrome coronavirus infections in camels.[36] An alternative approach that is being actively pursued for veterinary purposes is to use poxviruses, which have a more restricted host range. Much of this work has concentrated on the use of avipoxviruses, in particular, fowlpox and canarypox, as vectors for various veterinary species. These have been successfully exploited for several diseases, including Newcastle disease, avian influenza, equine influenza, rabies, FeLV, and canine distemper.[37,38] Other poxviruses that have been studied as veterinary vaccine vectors include capripox virus for rinderpest, racoonpox for rabies, parapox for pseudorabies, suipox for swine influenza, and myxomavirus for rabbit hemorrhagic disease.[35,39] Veterinary herpes viruses (eg, infectious bovine rhinotracheitis virus, feline herpes virus, and pseudorabies virus) and adenoviruses (eg, canine, equine, avian, and chimpanzee adenovirus) are also being developed as vectors. One particularly notable example is the herpesvirus of turkeys, which has been particularly successfully applied as a vector within the poultry industry for bivalent vaccines against Marek disease and IBR, IBD, or NDV.[40] In addition, a commercial trivalent vector vaccine has recently been developed against Marek, NDV, and IBD.[41]

2. Bacterial vectors: Recent studies on the rational attenuation of bacteria in order to produce suitable safe oral vaccines have introduced the possibility of using the vaccine strains generated as live vectors for foreign proteins. Majority of the

work in this area has concentrated on producing invasive strains of salmonella that are sufficiently attenuated so as not to cause any pathogenic disease symptoms when delivered orally to the host. Initial studies looked at generating auxotrophic mutants by removing or modifying important genes involved in the aromatic (aro) or purine (pur) synthesis pathways. Auxotrophic attenuation relies on the absence of the required nutrient in the host tissue, for example in the case of aro mutants the critical compounds are probably p-aminobenzoic acid and 2,4-dihydroxybenzoate. Both double aro and combination aro, pur mutants have been generated. Vaccination results are somewhat mixed; however, induction of local and systemic antibody and cell-mediated responses following oral immunization highlights the potential of this approach, and successful attenuated vaccines against salmonella in poultry have been produced.[42] Salmonella has also been used experimentally to vector several antigens, including *E coli*, *Shigella dysenteriae*, *Helicobacter pylori*, and transmissible gastroenteritis virus.[43] A further development in this field has come from studies into the use of Bacille Calmette-Guerin, a live attenuated bovine tubercle bacillus currently used to immunize humans against tuberculosis, as a vector. This mycobacterium is known to be safe and immunogenic. Furthermore, it can be given as a single oral dose; it is fairly heat stable, and it is inexpensive to produce. As a result, it has been engineered for overexpression homologous Ag85b as well as heterologous *E coli* and enterovirus 71 proteins. Other potential bacterial vectors include *Vibrio cholera*, *Yersinia enterocolitica*, *Listeria monocytogenes*, *Lactobacillus casei*, and *Streptococcus gordonii*.[44]

3. Protozoal vectors: One further and highly novel vector technology is based on the use of a live protozoan parasite (*Eimeria*) that has been genetically modified to deliver homologous or heterologous antigens to poultry. Such vaccines would use the currently licensed commercial attenuated strains that have been developed to vaccinate chickens against coccidiosis. Foreign genes would be expressed within the attenuated vectors using enzyme-mediated integration. The resultant transgenic strains could then be delivered in order to provide broader protection against coccidiosis infections or dual protection against coccidiosis and another infectious disease of chickens. The proof of concept for this approach has recently been reported by engineering a modified strain of *Eimeria tenella* to deliver the CjA protein of Campylobacter. This recombinant vaccine has been shown to provide between 86% and 91% immune protection against *Campylobacter jejuni* challenge when compared with unvaccinated and wild-type *E tenella* vaccinated controls ($P<.001$).[45]

Nucleic Acid Vaccines

A relatively new vaccine technology that falls between live and killed approaches is the nucleic acid vaccine. These vaccines are based on DNA cloned into a delivery plasmid or the direct injection of messenger RNA. They can be produced cost-effectively, and the endogenous protein synthesis mimics a natural infection. Thus, the antigens are presented in their native form and will elicit both MHC class I and class II T-cell responses as well as an antibody response. In addition, there is no risk of infection, and these vaccines can be used to bypass passive immunity.[46] The first licensed applications of this technology in 2005 were for the control of infectious hematopoietic necrosis virus disease in Canadian Atlantic salmon[47] and for the control of West Nile virus in horses.[48] DNA vaccines have also been licensed in Europe for salmon pancreas disease.[49]

SUMMARY

The field of veterinary vaccination has seen many significant advances in technologies over the past 25 years, with the introduction of several vaccines based on novel recombinant DNA technology. Such vaccines are designed to offer the farmer, owner, and clinician safer and more efficacious alternatives to existing vaccine technologies. In addition, they can have the added advantage of ease of administration and improved stability. Indeed, many new vaccine technologies often find their first commercial application within veterinary medicine, and, with the current interest in One Health approaches to humans, animals, and the environment, veterinary vaccines have an important role to play in the development of novel approaches. This article has covered some of the many new inactivated/killed and attenuated/live vaccination strategies that are now available to the veterinary research worker. A great deal more still needs to be understood about the nature of the responses required to elicit full protective immunity to several diseases. This knowledge should enable the development and construction of new generations of vaccines with more defined properties. It is already apparent that veterinary medicine will play a key role in such developments, and it is clear that this very active research area offers a great deal of potential for the development of further vaccine technologies in the future.

REFERENCES

1. Almeida JA, Brand C, Edwards DC, et al. Formation of virosomes from influenza subunits and liposomes. Lancet 1975;2:899–901.
2. Morein B, Simons K. Subunit vaccines against enveloped viruses: virosomes, micelles and other protein complexes. Vaccine 1985;3:83–93.
3. Criscia E, Bárcenab J, Montoyaa M. Virus-like particle-based vaccines for animal viral infections. Inmunologia 2013;32:102–16.
4. Morein B, Sundquist B, Hogland S, et al. ISCOM, a novel structure for antigenic presentation of membrane proteins from enveloped viruses. Nature 1984;308: 457–60.
5. Mumford JA, Jessett DM, Rollinson EA, et al. Duration of protective efficacy of equine influenza immunostimulating complex/tetanus vaccines. Vet Rec 1994; 134:158–62.
6. Crouch CF, Daly J, Henley W, et al. The use of a systemic prime/mucosal boost strategy with an equine influenza ISCOM vaccine to induce protective immunity in horses. Vet Immunol Immunopath 2005;108:345–55.
7. Osterhaus A, Weijer K, Uytdehaag F, et al. Induction of protective immune response in cats by vaccination with feline leukaemia virus ISCOM. J Immunol 1985;135:591–6.
8. Schuuring C. New era vaccines. Nature 1982;296:792.
9. Marciani DJ, Kensil CR, Beltz GA, et al. Genetically-engineered subunit vaccine against feline leukaemia virus: protective immune response in cats. Vaccine 1991;9:89–96.
10. Gregg JM, Tschopp JF, Stillman C, et al. High level expression and assembly of hepatitis B surface antigen in the methylotrophic yeast Pistia pastoris. Bio/Technol 1987;5:479–85.
11. Martelli P, Ferrari L, Morganti M, et al. One dose of a porcine circovirus 2 subunit vaccine induces humoral and cell-mediated immunity and protects against porcine circovirus-associated disease under field conditions. Vet Microbiol 2011;149:339–51.

12. Uttenthala A, Le Potierb MF, Romeroc L, et al. Classical swine fever (CSF) marker vaccine trial I. Challenge studies in weaner pigs. Vet Microbiol 2001;83:85–106.

13. Thomas C, Young NJ, Judith H, et al. Evaluation of efficacy of mammalian and baculovirus expressed E2 subunit vaccine candidates to bovine viral diarrhea virus. Vaccine 2009;27:2387–93.

14. Hua RH, Huo H, Wang XL, et al. Generation and efficacy of recombinant classical swine fever virus E2 glycoprotein expressed in stable transgenic mammalian cell line. PLoS One 2014;9:1–9.

15. Hua RH, Li YN, Chen ZS, et al. Generation and characterization of a new mammalian cell line continuously expressing virus-like particles of Japanese encephalitis virus for a subunit vaccine candidate. BMC Biotechnol 2014;14:1–9.

16. Vermij P, Waltz F. USDA approves the first plant-based vaccine. Nat Biotech 2006;24:233–4.

17. Liew PS, Hair-Bejo M. Farming of plant-based veterinary vaccines and their applications for disease prevention in animals. Adv Virol 2015;936940:1–11.

18. Takeyama N, Kiyono H, Yuki Y. Plant-based vaccines for animals and humans: recent advances in technology and clinical trials. Ther Adv Vaccines 2015;3:139–54.

19. Langebeheim H, Arnon R, Sela M. Antiviral effect on MS-2 coliphage obtained with a synthetic antigen. Proc Natl Acad Sci USA 1976;73:4636–40.

20. Merrifield RB. Solid phase peptide synthesis. 1. the synthesis of a tetrapeptide. J Am Chem Soc 1963;85:2149–54.

21. Francis MJ. Peptide vaccines for viral diseases. Sci Prog 1990;74:115–30.

22. Bittle JL, Houghton RA, Alexander H, et al. Protection against foot and mouth disease by immunisation with a chemically synthesised peptide predicted from the viral nucleotide sequence. Nature 1982;298:30–3.

23. Di Marchi R, Brooke G, Gale G, et al. Protection of cattle against foot-and-mouth disease by a synthetic peptide. Science 1986;232:639–41.

24. Broekhuijsen MP, van Rijn JMM, Blom AJM, et al. Fusion proteins with multiple copies of the major antigenic determinant of foot-and-mouth disease virus protect both the natural host and laboratory animals. J Gen Virol 1987;68:3137–43.

25. Francis MJ. Synthetic peptides. Meth Mol Med 2003;87:115–31.

26. Francis MJ, Fry CM, Rowlands DJ, et al. Immune response to uncoupled peptides of foot-and-mouth disease virus. Immunology 1987;61:1–6.

27. Francis MJ, Hastings GZ, Syred AD, et al. Non-responsiveness to a foot-and-mouth disease virus peptide overcome by addition of foreign helper T-cell determinants. Nature 1987;330:168–70.

28. Francis MJ, Clarke BE. Peptide vaccines based on enhanced immunogenicity of peptide epitopes presented with T-cell determinants or hepatitis B core protein. Meth Enzymol 1989;178:659–75.

29. Wang CY, Chang TY, Walfield AM, et al. Effective synthetic peptide vaccine for foot-and-mouth disease in swine. Vaccine 2002;20:2603–10.

30. Broekhuijsen MP, Blom T, van Rijn J, et al. Synthesis of fusion proteins with multiple copies of antigenic determinant of foot-and-mouth disease virus. Gene 1986;49:189–97.

31. Francis MJ, Hastings GZ, Brown F, et al. Immunological evaluation of the multiple antigen peptide (MAP) system using a major immunogenic site of foot-and-mouth disease virus. Immunol 1991;73:249–54.

32. Clarke BE, Newton SE, Carroll AR, et al. Improved immunogenicity of a peptide epitope after fusion to hepatitis B core protein. Nature 1987;330:381–4.

33. Francis MJ. Use of hepatitis B core as a vehicle for presenting viral antigens. Rev Med Virol 1992;2:225–31.

34. Ganguly S, Padhy A, Para PA, et al. DIVA vaccines: a brief review on its novel facets for the eradication of infections of livestock and poultry. World J Clin Pharmacol Microbiol Toxicol 2015;1:22–3.
35. Sanchez-Sampedro L, Perdiguero B, Mejias-Perez E, et al. The evolution of poxvirus vaccines. Viruses 2015;7:1726–11803.
36. Haagmans BL, van den Brand JM, Raj VS, et al. An orthopoxvirus-based vaccine reduces virus excretion after MERS-CoV infection in dromedary camels. Science 2016;351:77–81.
37. Weli SC, Tryland M. Avipoxviruses: infection biology and their use as vaccine vectors. Virol J 2011;8:49–64.
38. Poulet H, Minke J, Pardo MC, et al. Development and registration of recombinant veterinary vaccines: the example of the canarypox vector platform. Vaccine 2007; 25:5606–12.
39. Spibey N, McCabe VJ, Greenwood NM, et al. Novel bivalent vectored vaccine for control of myxomatosis and rabbit haemorrhagic disease. Vet Rec 2012;170: 309–13.
40. Iqbal M. Progress toward the development of polyvalent vaccination strategies against multiple viral infections in chickens using herpesvirus of turkeys as vector. Bioengineered 2012;3:222–6.
41. Innovax-ND-IBD approval. Committee for Medicinal Products for Veterinary Use (CVMP) meeting. London, June 15, 2017.
42. Pei Y, Parreira VR, Roland KL, et al. Assessment of attenuated Salmonella vaccine strains in controlling experimental Salmonella typhimurium infection in chickens. Can J Vet Res 2014;78:23–30.
43. Rowland K, Brenneman KE. Salmonella as a vaccine delivery vehicle. Expert Rev Vaccin 2013;12:1033–45.
44. da Silva AJ, Zangirolami TC, Marques MT, et al. Live bacterial vaccine vectors: an overview. Braz J Microcbiol 2014;45:1117–29.
45. Clark JD, Oakes RD, Redhead K, et al. Eimeria species parasites as novel vaccine delivery vectors: anti-Campylobacter jejuni protective immunity induced by Eimeria tenella-delivered CjaA. Vaccine 2012;30:2683–8.
46. Donnelly JJ, Ulmer JB, Shiver JW, et al. DNA vaccines. Ann Rev Immunol 1997; 15:617–48.
47. Tonheim TC, Bøgwald J, Dalmo RA. What happens to the DNA vaccine in fish? A review of current knowledge. Fish Shellfish Immunol 2008;25:1–18.
48. Ledgerwood JE, Pierson TC, Hubka SA, et al. A West Nile virus DNA vaccine utilizing a modified promoter induces neutralizing antibody in younger and older healthy adults in a phase I clinical trial. J Infect Dis 2011;203:1396–404.
49. Evensen O, Leong J-A. DNA vaccines against viral diseases of farmed fish. Fish Shellfish Immunol 2013;35:1751–8.

Another Look at the "Dismal Science" and Jenner's Experiment

John A. Elllis, DVM, PhD

KEYWORDS

- Immunology • Adverse reactions • Memory • Vaccines

KEY POINTS

- Defense of the vertebrate body comprises 3 layers: physical barriers, innate immunity, adaptive immunity.
- B cells and antibodies recognize whole proteins; T cells recognize processed proteins.
- Innate immunity contributes to adverse reactions and vaccine efficacy.
- Overall effectiveness of vaccines and memory depends on the life style of the pathogen.

Immunology is a course that most veterinary students suffer through; many would consider its reappellation as the "dismal science" more than appropriate. One carrot in the course is the lectures on vaccines, because even a pedestrian pre-veterinary experience would indicate the continued relevance of the now 200 years plus-old gutsy, if not totally original, "experiment" of Edward Jenner[1]; vaccination remains a backbone of practice and the stuff of preventative medicine. The chapter on vaccines in immunology textbooks generally contains a table listing the advantages and disadvantages of live versus dead (inactivated) immunogens.[2] Live vaccines confer a broader, longer lasting immunity, require fewer doses, and are less likely to stimulate "hypersensitivity," whereas inactivated vaccines are stable and "safer" because they are less virulent and do not replicate in the vaccine. Beyond the midterm and final examinations in immunology class we have all internalized these "facts" at some level and consciously or unconsciously routinely apply them in practice. But, what features of the immune response and characteristics of pathogens and respective vaccines validate, or invalidate, our working assumptions? How does an understanding of the basic science of "vaccinology" avert oversimplification, thereby avoiding unrealistic

Disclosure: The author has conducted funded vaccine efficacy studies for most veterinary biologics firms, including: Zoetis, Wyeth Animal Health, Fort Dodge, Merial, Boehringer-Ingelheim, and Elanco.
Department of Veterinary Microbiology, Western College of Veterinary Medicine, University of Saskatchewan, 52 Campus Drive, Saskatoon, Saskatchewan S7N 5B4, Canada
E-mail address: john.ellis@usask.ca

expectations of vaccine efficacy and duration of immunity, and misunderstandings regarding "adverse reactions" (to vaccines)? And, how do more recent studies in the dismal science broaden our understanding and suggest further applications for vaccination? This review is an attempt to again address this subject for the practicing small animal veterinarian; hopefully, being both at least somewhat practical, and not overly soporific.

A BRIEF OVERVIEW OF THE "DISMAL SCIENCE": IMMUNOLOGY

Conceptually, defense of the vertebrate body can be seen to consist of 3 overlapping layers. The first layer comprises constitutive anatomy, microanatomy, and physiology. The skin, the body's largest organ, is the most obvious example of a physical barrier. Ciliated epithelium and the overlying "mucous," that is actually a complex cocktail, comprise the "mucociliary escalator" that perform housekeeping functions in the respiratory tract.[3,4] A similar microanatomical/physiologic barrier is found in the gastrointestinal tract.[5] These barriers keep the respective mucosal surfaces "scrubbed" of pathogens. In recent years, the microbiota or "normal flora" of various body systems, especially the mucosae, have been much studied as a modulator of colonization by pathogens.[3,4,6] All of these protective constitutive structures and functions can be affected by a variety of co-factors ranging from poor nutrition to the number of air changes in a boarding kennel, thereby precluding the possibility that vaccination can be the "silver bullet" solution to every (management) problem.[4,7]

If the constitutive barriers are breached by pathogenic microbes, the next layer, the innate immune response, comes into play. Although innate immunity has long been recognized as an ancient part of vertebrate defenses,[8] it is only in the last couple of decades that it has been intensively studied, more fully characterized, and taught to any extent in veterinary curricula. The plethora of molecular interactions that comprise the innate immune response is perhaps best summarily thought of as an inflammatory response involving a variety of cells that are spread throughout the body, including neutrophils, eosinophils, natural killer cells, and monocytes and macrophages; soluble mediators, notably type I interferons; and the often memorized and forgotten cascade, complement.[9-11] Traditionally, innate immune responses have been considered to be "nonspecific" and devoid of "memory."

If invaders persist in defiance of an innate immune response, adaptive or acquired immune responses are triggered; that part of the overall response that medical professionals have generally paid most attention to, because it is these responses that have been traditionally associated with the use of vaccines. Even the most immunophobic of veterinarians, of course, remember that the adaptive response comprises both "humoral" or antibody responses involving B lymphocytes and plasma cells, and cell-mediated immunity responses involving acronym-shrouded, too complicated subpopulations of T lymphocytes and the cytokines they produce.[12] Historically, specificity and memory differentiate adaptive responses versus innate responses.

HOW DOES THE IMMUNE SYSTEM "SEE THE WORLD," AND WHAT ARE THE IMPLICATIONS FOR VACCINE CHOICE AND EFFICACY?

As with all the rest of life on the planet, interactions between the immune system and the outside world unavoidably, ultimately, come down to biochemical reactions; in this case receptor-ligand interactions, a common modus operandi in most body systems. Generically, in the case of the innate response, the ligands are biochemical motifs or patterns that are "foreign"; not found in vertebrates. Notable examples include endotoxin (lipopolysaccharide), negative-stranded RNA, and bacterial DNA.[13] These are commonly known as "danger signals" or more technically, pathogen-associated molecular patterns (PAMPs). Beginning with Toll-like receptors, a dizzying array of other receptors that are biochemically arranged into families such as NOD and RAG are now recognized. They are generically lumped as pattern recognition receptors (PRRs). The PRRs electrostatically bind their ligands, danger signals; some PRRs are expressed on the cell membrane, whereas others are found intracellularly.[13,14]

In contrast, the ligands for most protective adaptive responses are bits of protein, called "epitopes" or antigenic determinants.[15] Some of these are linear epitopes, based on the primary structure of proteins; in other words, the simple linear arrangement of amino acids that make up a protein; others are "conformational" epitopes or determinates based on the secondary, tertiary, or quaternary structure of proteins, or the overall arrangement of amino acids based on the way proteins are folded. The latter can be particularly sensitive to alteration by inactivation processes.[12,15]

Beyond differences in receptor–ligand interactions, the 2 major players in adaptive immunity, B and T lymphocytes, see the world in very different ways. Essentially, B cells and antibodies, whether "fixed" on the cell surface as receptors, or when secreted and acting as effector molecules, interact with epitopes on whole proteins, whereas T cells interact with epitopes from "processed" proteins.[16–19] This conceptual detail goes a long way to explaining the types of pathogens or stages of infection that are likely to be most susceptible to which type of response, B cells and antibodies versus T cells, and, ultimately what type of vaccine is likely to be most effective against what pathogen. For example, antibodies can be very effective at neutralizing bacterial toxins (secreted proteins) in tissue spaces, or viruses (through interaction with their surface proteins) that are shed on mucosal surfaces; in other words, by recognizing epitopes comprising intact proteins from/on extracellular invaders. In contrast "killer" T lymphocytes can eradicate cells that are already infected with a virus or intracellular bacterium based on the recognition of a foreign epitope presented on the surface of the infected cell; in other words, "bits" of foreign proteins that derive from "processing" of the constituents of pathogens within the infected cell. Similarly, "helper" T cells will secrete cytokines such as interleukin (IL)-2 or IL-4, or important new ones that you may not have heard of, such as IL-17,[20] in response to "seeing" a foreign epitope on a "professional" antigen-presenting cell, notably one of the many types of dendritic cells.[21] Inevitably, differences in T-cell functions relate to differences in antigen presentation to the respective T cells in the context of the infamous major histocompatibility complex (MHC) molecules.[18,19] Killer T cells see foreign epitopes presented in the "folds" of MHC-I molecules that are expressed on virtually all cells of the body (except, notably, red blood cells). This property allows the killer T cells to perform "search and destroy" missions in all body systems; any cell that is infected can process viral, bacterial, or parasite proteins and shuttle resultant peptides to the cell surface; therefore, any cell can be a target for destruction. In contrast, helper T cells see foreign epitopes together with MHC-II molecules, which are restricted in their expression, notably to antigen-presenting cells that take up and process foreign proteins.[19,20,22]

So then, what possible usefulness is there in reconjuring this immunologic dogma? Regurgitating and understanding these basic tenets elucidates informed vaccine selection, based on the "lifestyle" of a particular pathogen, extracellular versus intracellular. For example, some of the oldest and still most effective vaccines in human and veterinary medicine are "toxids," or inactivated toxins. When these fixed whole proteins are injected, B lymphocytes are triggered, and plasma cells make antibodies to numerous epitopes comprising these proteins. Similarly, inactivated bacterial vaccines or "bacterins" of various sorts, as well as more modern subunit formulations, present the adaptive immune system with proteins resulting in production of neutralizing antibodies. Historically, and currently these types of responses, whether used actively in the vaccinated individual or used passively for therapy, can result in disease-sparing and life-saving outcomes in a variety of bacterial infections such as those caused by *Clostridium spp* or *Bordetella spp.*[23] But, in contrast, similarly formulated, and traditionally adjuvanted (eg, Alum) inactivated viral vaccines do not prime for protective killer T-lymphocyte responses, simply because they do not result in "infection" of cells, thereby precluding natural processing and antigen presentation of viral peptides on a cell surface together with MHC-I molecules. For the latter to occur, a (modified) live virus or live, gene-carrying vector, such as canary pox, is required for the "endogenous" pathway of antigen presentation. However, inactivated viral (and bacterial) vaccines can stimulate cytokine secretion of, for example, interferon-gamma, by helper T cells as a result of phagocytosis or pinocytosis of vaccine by an antigen-presenting cells, processing of "ingested" proteins, and appearance of peptides in the context of MHC-II molecules on the cell surface; peptides that a helper T cell can "see." This possibility partially explains the observed efficacy of some inactivated viral vaccines, even if killer T lymphocytes are not primed for. Conversely, similar processing via this "exogenous" pathway can also occur with live vaccines, resulting in the secretion of cytokines that "help" the overall response to a pathogen. The latter more holistic subtleties of cell-mediated immunity are often overlooked in a strict dichotomous view of live versus inactivated vaccines.

THAT WHICH DOES NOT KILL US, MAKES US STRONGER: ANOTHER LOOK AT "ADVERSE REACTIONS" TO VACCINATION

A predictable, but nonetheless ironic, consequence of the overall success of vaccination in human and veterinary medicine is the current focus on "adverse reactions" to vaccination; a focus on the rare trees versus the forest. What is usually lost in the alternative facts of this, in addition to the actual low prevalence and incidence of adverse responses to vaccination in pet populations, overall[24,25] is a misunderstanding of the mechanisms responsible for most adverse reactions; "hypersensitivity," particularly type I hypersensitivity, is usually implicated. In the landmark studies of Moore and colleagues[24] conducted more than a decade ago, it was documented that little dogs that received multiple vaccines (usually including a bacterial vaccine) on the same visit had the highest incidence of adverse reactions. Do these data imply that "little dogs" are more "allergic"? Certainly, allergic reactions of various sorts, often genetically associated, are responsible for some adverse reactions.[26] But, what these data more likely elucidate in the case of most dogs, regardless of size, with swelling, soreness, fever, malaise, inappetence, and so on, after vaccination is the "double-edged sword" of innate immunity. First, injecting the same amount of "danger signals" (PAMPs) into a small body, compared with a large body, is more likely to cause proinflammatory cytokine "intoxication"; it is a dose effect, most often observable in small dogs and cats.[24,27] This intoxication, most likely, is the physiologic basis of most reported adverse reactions. But, on the other side of the sword, one of the many intricacies of the overall immune response that is often forgotten as immunology class gets further away in the rear-view mirror is the "overlap" in innate and adaptive immune responses.[28,29] Simply put, some of the same soluble mediators, proinflammatory cytokines such as IL-1 and IL-6, are a necessary bridge between innate and adaptive immunity. Essentially, without some level of inflammation in the response to a vaccine, memory is not effectively established.[30] Taking this beyond just more immunologic "theory" is the experience with vaccines for whooping cough (*Bordetella pertussis*) in humans, with good epidemiologic evidence supporting the concept that, although no longer used, whole cell *B pertussis* bacterins were more "reactogenic" than currently used subunit vaccines,[31] they apparently conferred more durable immunity.[31,32] There is some evidence that a similar disparity in immunogenicity applies to whole cell versus acellular *Bordetella bronchiseptica* vaccines for dogs as well.[33,34] Relatedly, individuals who survive the widespread viral replication and associated inflammation of morbillivirus infections (measles or canine distemper virus)[35,36] are likely to have more durable immunity than individuals that are vaccinated with attenuated viruses, especially if never exposed to field viruses because of good herd immunity in highly vaccinated populations.[37] Conversely, administration of intranasal vaccines containing respiratory pathogens that replicate only locally and cause little inflammation can result in immunity of relatively short duration (months) if not boosted naturally or iatrogenically.[38]

In summary, concerning innate immunity (inflammation) in the context of vaccination, perhaps it is best to think like Goldilocks. What is desirable is an accompanying innate response that is not too strong and not too weak, but an elusive just right (amount). Without this just right amount, less than optimal (adaptive) immunity occurs, whereas with too much of it, adverse reactions of variable severity occur. From a practical standpoint, in human medicine, prevaccination treatment with antiinflammatory (analgesic) drugs, specifically, aspirin or acetaminophen, has been used successfully as prophylaxis in some patients, especially those with a history of pronounced adverse reactions to vaccination. Use of these drugs is obviously not possible in small animals, owing to species-determined toxicities. Although more specifically acting, generally nontoxic, nonsteroidal antiinflammatory drugs that target the cyclooxygenase 2 pathway are available in veterinary medicine, at least for dogs, there is some evidence that inhibition of cyclooxygenase 2 (including by aspirin) may not only decrease pain and other symptoms of adverse reactions, but also decrease immune (antibody) responses as well,[39] making it problematic to recommend such drugs in a similar prophylactic application before vaccination of pets. Until such time when evidence-based pharmacologic intervention can be justified, reduction in the numbers of doses of vaccines given simultaneously is warranted in patients with a history of adverse reactions to vaccines.[24] In other words, apply the art of practice in modulating the innate immune response.

LIKE DÉJÀ VU ALL OVER AGAIN: THE PROMISE AND LIMITATIONS OF IMMUNOLOGIC MEMORY

Innate immune responses have evolved to have spatial and temporal boundaries; they are meant to be short lived and targeted. Illustrative of the importance of these constraints is the pathophysiology that results from unremitting stimulation of innate immunity in the case of chronic infections, such as with *Mycobacteria ssp.*,[40] or the tricky business of achieving a therapeutic versus pathologic result after iatrogenic systemic dosing of interferons or other proinflammatory cytokines.[41] Relatedly, the traditional view of the innate immune response presupposes a lack of memory, thereby precluding an immunologic déjà vu when it comes to "experiencing" danger signals, but also averting cytokine intoxication owing to anamnestic responses. In other words, every time a vertebrate "sees" endotoxin, it is like the first time from the standpoint of an innate immune response to it. Or, so it was thought. Then, in 2011, Netea and colleagues[42] thinking laterally and considering old data from classical mammalian immunology,[43] and more recent data from invertebrate[44] and plant[45] "immunology" proposed the idea of "trained (innate) immunity." In essence, they defined the memory of trained immunity as a heightened response to secondary infection that can be exerted both toward the same microorganism or a different one (cross-protection).[42] The response cannot be defined as either strictly innate (because it is induced only secondarily in hosts that have been previously exposed or vaccinated) nor adaptive (because it is independent of the epitopic specificity of T- and B-cell responses).[42] The mechanisms that mediate the heightened activation state involves cells such as macrophages and natural killer cells, entails improved pathogen recognition by PRRs, and, ultimately, an enhanced protective inflammatory response.[42]

Currently, there are no formal studies that have specifically addressed this concept in domestic animals; nevertheless, there are at least several implications and applications related to thinking about "trained (innate) immunity" for the practicing veterinarian. Ironically, ever since the decades-old documentation that intranasal delivery of herpesvirus can stimulate production of (type I) interferon,[46] many veterinarians, mostly on the cow side of the black bag, have been taking advantage of trained innate immunity for years through the practice of intranasal vaccination of high-risk animals, or a population of animals in the face of an outbreak. In this application, they have been ahead of our colleagues in human medicine. Now there is a better, but not complete, understanding about why this can be disease sparing; it is beyond a simple type I interferon response, and fits the bill of trained innate immunity. For example, a commonly used 3-way intranasal viral vaccine in calves containing respiratory syncytial virus, herpesvirus, and parainfluenza virus not only contains many specific epitopes that stimulate the adaptive immune system, it also contains many danger signals or PAMPs that will interact with multiple PRRs and stimulate innate immune responses that can not only effect these viruses upon infection, but also potentially modulate infections with unrelated pathogens. Similarly, although not commonly thought of or used in this way, administering a 3-way intranasal vaccine containing B bronchiseptica, parainfluenza virus and adenovirus to dogs (or cats) will not only trigger adaptive immune responses to these pathogens, but also trigger innate immune pathways that could reduce disease in kenneled or otherwise commingled pets. Some experimental data support the application of this concept in small animals. Cats that were given a 2-way intranasal vaccine containing calicivirus and herpesvirus had less disease than unvaccinated controls when they were subsequently challenged with B bronchiseptica, implying a disease-sparing "cross-protective" innate or trained immune response.[47] In addition to its progressive, if now obvious, application with intranasal vaccines, there is mounting evidence from experimental studies and clinical trials in human medicine of similar effects after the administration of parenteral vaccines, particularly commonly used "whole organism" vaccines such as BCG, measles, influenza, and yellow fever.[48,49] Although still under investigation, intuitively, the wide range of PAMPs in these formulations (compared with subunit vaccines) are likely to be implicated mechanistically. It is early days in this field; however, this means stimulating cross-protective responses to pathogens for which there are currently no vaccines provides a further application and justification for routine vaccination of pets with currently available combination vaccines that are already in widespread use.

As mentioned, it is important to consider the double-edged sword when tweaking the innate immune system iatrogenically. If an animal's innate immune response is already upregulated by, for example, a subclinical infection, adding more inflammatory cytokines to the system could tip the balance from protection to pathology. Again, a place for the art of practice.

Traditionally, the hallmarks of adaptive immunity have been considered to be specificity and memory. We all learned this. We also learned about "memory cells" that expand to make more B and T cells that effectuate more rapid and efficient responses in vaccinated or previously exposed animals. From a mechanistic standpoint, immune memory has been a much-studied area that nevertheless remains unresolved and controversial. It is still largely a "black box," more complicated than choosing answer "D" (memory cells) on a multiple choice test, and beyond the scope of this review. Suffice it to say that what is perceived as immune memory comprises some combination of, at least, classical "memory cells," long-lived plasma cells and persistence of antigen.[50-55] Vaccine recommendations and practical experience tell us that this varies among vaccines.

Beyond the mechanics of memory, the pathogenesis of various infections, in other words the "lifestyle" of individual pathogens, plays a significant role in affecting vaccine efficacy and having, and conveying to, clients' realistic expectations for vaccine efficacy.[54-56] In both human and veterinary medicine, there has been a tendency to formulate and use combination versus single component vaccines. From a practical standpoint, this makes sense; contributing to overall convenience and reducing the number of "needles" a child or a pet receives, a laudable goal as part of placating anti-vaccinationists. Some of the most commonly used immunogens in small medicine are exemplary of this approach; notably "DAPP" for dogs and "FVRCP" for cats. However, they are also exemplary, in many cases, of overly great expectations for vaccine efficacy overall. Generically, pathogens that have a complicated lifestyles and resultant long incubation or prodromal period, owing to, for example, an obligatory phase of amplified replication in lymphoid tissues before proceeding back to mucosal surfaces, are more effectively controlled by vaccination, because the lag period between infection and disease allows for classical memory cell populations to expand into effector cell populations.[54-56] Thankfully, some of the main microbial killers of people and their animals fit this pattern and can be very effectively controlled or eradicated with vaccination; because the immune response wins the "race" with the pathogen. Small pox virus, morbilliviruses (measles, canine distemper virus), carnivore parvoviruses, and adenoviruses (canine infectious hepatitis) have this lifestyle, and vaccines, and resultant memory (cell) responses, for these can provide robust and long-lived immunity. Other pathogens ranging in virulence form parainfluenza viruses and *B bronchiseptica* to filoviruses (Ebola virus) cause disease at the site of entry without systemic replication or replicate very rapidly, and can essentially "outrun" a memory response, requiring higher levels of effector functions at the time of infection for optimal or any disease sparing.[54-56] Similarly, bacterial infections that tend toward persistence and chronicity, notably *Borrelia spp* and *Leptospira spp,* probably also require higher effector function and near sterilizing immunity at the time of exposure to prevent the establishment of infection by low numbers of bacteria that survive lower levels of antibody at increasing times from vaccination. This usually means more frequent vaccination. Ironically, and similar to the history of vaccines for *B pertussis*, the newer generation of vaccines for these pathogens, although considerably less reactive and "smoother" are probably, although comparatively untested, relatively less effective at stimulating the production of protective antibody as well. In other words, you cannot always have the immunologic cake and eat it too. These examples are illustrative of the disparity possible between being "immune" (ie, having some measurable memory or effector function) and being "protected."[54,56,57] The plot thickens even further when considering the strategies that some pathogens have evolved to evade the immune response, including adaptive memory. RNA viruses in general are highly mutable. We all learned this. Exemplary of such a "mutation machine" is feline calicivirus (FCV), which has been elegantly shown to evolve in real time in multicat households.[58] From a practical standpoint, what this means is that although FCV vaccines, usually containing 1 isolate of the virus, induce antibody responses that cross-react among genetically divergent FCV isolates, immunity is incomplete, and the virus can persist, evolve, and cause disease even in vaccinated cats.[59] Alpha herpesviruses, for example, feline herpesvirus, have a different survival scheme and are endemic in their respective host populations, almost always resulting in latent infections, but are relatively invariable, antigenically. We all learned this. So that, even a well-vaccinated cat, even one living alone with a primate with its own species-specific herpesvirus, can get clinical feline herpesvirus "infection" again and again without seeing another cat when latent virus recrudesces. Those minority of us nearly universally herpesvirus simplex latently infected primates who get "cold sores" can immediately relate. So, the frustrated experienced owner with a new kitten, expecting "sterile immunity" asks, "Why vaccinate?" It is simple, if not overt without an unvaccinated control: disease associated with FCV or feline herpesvirus infections will usually be reduced, that is, "less severe," in the vaccinated cat, thanks largely to the establishment of "memory," and improvement (boosting) of memory and effector functions by routine vaccination (antigen exposure). From another one health (perspective), a topical and relevant vindication of the latter concept is the demonstrated efficacy of, and recommendations for, the new shingles (ie, herpes zoster) vaccine for the aging primate pet owner.[60] As in an adult cat getting FRCVP, it boosts on board "memory" responses to the latent herpesvirus. The anamnestic response curtails viral replication, thereby reducing disease, if not eliminating the infection. Admittedly, the devil in all of these details would make the majority of clients snore, but are important to understanding the limitations of (adaptive) immune memory, why the "efficacy" of responses to all the pathogens contained in the same bottle of DAPP or FRCVP will not necessarily be the same, and why some vaccines need to be given more frequently than others.

Dovetailing with any discussion of immune memory is a consideration of duration of immunity, which has been part and parcel to the "vaccine debate" since its inception, and now has become central to any (intelligent) discussion about "titer testing." There have been many study reports and reviews written concerning duration of immunity of veterinary vaccines, and referencing and extensive discussing of the topic is beyond the scope of this review, except to say that at least one elephant in the room is the virtual absence of critical population data beyond titers. In other words, essentially, there has been scant, at best, meaningful association made between titers, and clinical outcomes in properly vaccinated pet populations outside of laboratories. Certainly, serology, that is, "titer testing," has been and is central to assessing vaccine efficacy and duration of immunity in human medicine.[61] But, that is where similarity (with veterinary medicine) ends, as it has generally not been resulting from a plethora of unstandardized tests and methodologies. More important, even though physicians have not generally had the "luxury" of experimentally challenging vaccinees, there has been a large infrastructure and resources to monitor disease outcomes in large populations, even if in some cases the ethics of clinical trials have been questionable.[62] Together, the data have allowed the determination of actual amounts of antibody that are correlated with protection from naturally acquired clinical disease in the case of many important human infections.[61,62] In contrast, it can be at the same time entertaining and depressingly illuminating to query various commercial entities that perform "titer testing" in small animals as to what their "protective titers" are actually based on; there is often (stunned) silence on the other end of the line. Summarily, from the standpoint of current reality, the coming tsunami of demands for titer testing in our profession is, arguably, reminiscent of Dorothy's return trip to Kansas. It sounds good in principle, but when one looks behind the wizards' curtains, it is less than convincing that the promised outcome can be delivered.

Acknowledging, or not, the gestalt of duration of immunity and the complexity of its assessment at the population level, perhaps it is instructive to consider one common and often frustrating example related to duration of immunity: 1-year versus 3-year rabies vaccines. Rabies virus and vaccines for it are almost unique in veterinary medicine, given the obvious public health issues. It, therefore, represents a best case scenario for a standardized approach to the assessment of vaccine efficacy and duration of immunity in our profession. First, for peace of mind, it is important to acknowledge that in many if not most cases in North America the mandated frequency of vaccination for rabies, that is, a de facto assessment of duration of immunity, is determined by jurisdictional fiat, not data. Otherwise, how could adjoining localities have different requirements for use of the same or similar vaccines?[63] It is akin to airport security; it is the law, get over it. A more logical law is the readily Internet-accessible (United States) code of federal regulations ("9-CFR") concerning the licensing of rabies vaccines, both live and killed.[64,65] There is detailed description of testing criteria involving a stringent challenge using an experimental method of transmission (intramuscular) that mimics the natural mode. Simply put, if a manufacturer seeks a 3-year label claim, vaccinees (and controls) need to be challenged, and pass the test, 3 years after vaccination. This of course allows for the possibility that there may be little if any difference(s) between a vaccine that is licensed for 3 years (between boosters) and 1 year, other than in the latter case the manufacturer did not go through the time, money, and logistics to challenge the requisite number of vaccinated dogs and/or cats at 3 years after vaccination. That aside, what do we know about protective immunity in rabies virus infections? We all learned about the pathogenesis of rabies virus infection; it is been known for a long time, with more recent studies simply adding interesting details around the edges.[66] It is a classic, with some local virus replication in muscle at the site of a bite, a relatively rapid entry into axons at synapses, retrograde travel to the brain, and an obituary a variable time thereafter. Predictably, there is a large literature around rabies vaccines and the immune responses there to, including the complexity of the response,[63,66] which warrants its own review. This complexity, involving cell-mediated immunity, is the stuff of the caveat emptor that just because an animal does not have a (rabies) "titer" does not mean it is not protected.[63] But, a more important, if less frequently communicated, caveat emptor is the almost certain variation in response to rabies virus vaccines, including such factors as animal age, size (smaller dogs usually develop higher titers), and inconsistencies in (licensed) vaccine immunogenicity.[67] And, a smaller less read and cited literature concerning people and animals that survive rabies virus infection is arguably more elucidative of the Ockham's razor of protective immunity in rabies virus infections.[68] Animals that do not have a systemic "high" virus-neutralizing antibody titer that is readily measurable in serum at the time of exposure have a poor prognosis, period. This is predictable by remembering pathogenesis of the infection.[54,56,66] Whatever vaccine(s) or (boosting) protocol that results in this outcome in the majority of vaccinees should be recommended and (titer) tested for. These observations also question the role/true efficacy of the recommended boosting of adaptive immunity after exposure[63] given the time required for an anamnestic antibody response, and the less than likely exposure of the virus to that antibody once in the immunologically privileged site of the axon (and the central nervous system). Moreover, this bottom line of protection (vs mere immunity) supports the practice of passive immunization, as soon as possible, as part of postexposure management in humans,[69] and begs the question, why is this not done in postexposure management of dogs and cats, especially because there is the recommendation for postexposure management in the bitee in any case where the biter is suspect (of being rabid) anyway?[69] Regardless of some apparent inconsistencies in rules around its use, routine vaccination against rabies virus has been a significant success story in veterinary medicine and also impacts, big time, zoonotic transmission, as best evidenced by its absence in many parts of the world.[63]

SUMMARY

The follow-up to Jenner's experiment, routine vaccination, has reduced more disease and saved more vertebrate lives than any other iatrogenic procedure by orders of magnitude. The unassailability of that potentially provocative cliché has been ciphered in human medicine, even if it is more difficult to do in our profession. It is also cliché to say that it is not "100%" (effective) and is not without "risk"; in those ways, it is consistent with life in general. It would seem that the bulk of the public relations headaches concerning vaccines in practice are the result of a "failure to communicate," often resulting in overly great expectations among clientele. All that to say and propose that, even in the throes of a tight appointment schedule remembering and synopsizing (for clients) some details of the dismal science can make practice great again.

REFERENCES

1. Turk JL, Allen E. The influence of John Hunter's inoculation practice on Edward Jenner's discovery of vaccination against smallpox. J R Soc Med 1990;83(4): 266–7.
2. Tizard IR. Vaccines and their production. In: Tizard IR, editor. Veterinary immunology. 9th edition. St Louis (MO): Elsevier, Inc; 2013. p. 258–71.
3. Ackermann MR, Derscheid R, Roth JA. Innate immunology of bovine respiratory disease. Vet Clin North Am Food Anim Pract 2010;26:215–28.
4. Caswell JL. Failure of respiratory defenses in the pathogenesis of bacterial pneumonia in cattle. Vet Pathol 2014;51(2):393–409.
5. Mason KL, Huggnagle GB. Control of mucosal polymicrobial populations by innate immunity. Cell Microbiol 2009;11(9):1297–305.
6. Denny JE, Powell WL, Schmidt NW. Local and long-distance calling: conversations between gut microbiota and intra- and extra gastrointestinal tract infections. Front Cell Infect Microbiol 2016;6:1–9.
7. Jonkers DM. Microbial perturbations and modulation in conditions associated with malnutrition and malabsorption. Best Pract Res Clin Gastroenterol 2016; 30(2):161–72.
8. Ward AE, Rosenthal BM. Evolutionary responses of innate to adaptive immunity. Infect Genet Evol 2014;21:492–6.
9. Wonjo T, Artis D. Emerging concepts and future challenges in innate lymphoid cell biology. J Exp Med 2016;213(11):2229–48.
10. Liu J, Cao X. Cellular and molecular regulation of innate inflammatory responses. Cell Mol Immunol 2016;13:711–21.
11. Freeley S, Kemper C, Le Friec G. The "ins and outs" of complement-driven immune responses. Immunol Rev 2016;274(1):16–32.
12. Nicholson LB. The immune system. Essays Biochem 2016;60:275–301.
13. Akira S, Uematsu S, Takeuchi O. Pathogen recognition and innate immunity. Cell 2006;124:783–801.
14. Kawai T, Akira S. Toll-like receptors and their crosstalk with other innate receptors of infection and immunity. Immunity 2011;34:637–50.
15. Floudas CA, Fung HK, McAllister SR, et al. Advances in protein structure prediction and de novo protein design: a review. Chem Engin Sci 2006;61:966–88.

16. Livingstone AM, Fathman CG. The structure of T-cell epitopes. Annu Rev Immunol 1987;5:477–510.
17. Batista FD, Harwood NE. The who, how and where of antigen presentation to B cells. Nat Rev Immunol 2009;9:15–27.
18. Blander JM. The comings and goings of MHC class I molecules herald a new dawn in cross-presentation. Immunol Rev 2016;272(1):65–79.
19. Bretou M, Kumari A, Malbec O, et al. Dynamics of the membrane –cytoskeleton interface in MHC class II-restricted antigen presentation. Immunol Rev 2016; 272(1):39–51.
20. Miossec P, Korn T, Kuchroo VK. Interleukin-17 and type 17 helper cells. N Engl J Med 2009;361:888–98.
21. Patel VI, Metcalf JP. Identification and characterization of human dendritic cell subsets in the steady state: a review of our current knowledge. J Investig Med 2016;64(4):833–47.
22. Jakubzick CV, Randolph GJ, Henson PM. Monocyte differentiation and antigen-presenting functions. Nat Rev Immunol 2017;17(6):349–62.
23. Casdevall A, Dadachova E, Pirofski LA. Passive antibody therapy for infectious diseases. Nat Rev Microbiol 2004;2:695–703.
24. Moore GE, Guptill LF, Ward MP, et al. Adverse events diagnosed within three days of vaccine administration in dogs. J Am Vet Med Assoc 2005;227(7):1102–8.
25. Moore GE, DeSantis-Kerr AC, Guptill LF, et al. Adverse events after vaccine administration in cats: 2,560 cases (2002-2005). J Am Vet Med Assoc 2007; 231(1):94–100.
26. Moore GE, HogenEsch H. Adverse vaccinal events in dogs and cats. Vet Clin North Am Small Anim Pract 2010;40:393–407.
27. Starr RM. Reaction rate in cats vaccinated with a new controlled-titer feline pan-leukopenia-rhinotracheitis-calicivirus-*chlamydia psittaci* vaccine. Cornell Vet 1993;83(4):311–23.
28. Kang SM, Compans RW. Host responses from innate to adaptive immunity after vaccination: molecular and cellular events. Mol Cells 2009;27(1):5–14.
29. Iwasaki A, Medzhitov R. Regulation of adaptive immunity by the innate immune system. Science 2010;327(5963):291–5.
30. Castellino F, Galli G, Del Giudice G, et al. Generating memory with vaccination. Eur J Immunol 2009;39(8):2100–5.
31. Mattoo S, Cherry JD. Molecular pathogenesis, epidemiology, and clinical manifestations of respiratory infections due to *Bordetella pertussis* and other *Bordetella* subspecies. Clin Microbiol Rev 2005;18(2):326–82.
32. Sealey KL, Belcher T, Preston A. *Bordetella pertussis* epidemiology and evolution in the light of pertussis resurgence. Infect Genet Evol 2016;40:136–43.
33. Ellis JA, Krakowka GS, Dayton AD, et al. Comparative efficacy of an injectable vaccine and an intranasal vaccine in stimulating *Bordetella bronchiseptica*-reactive antibody responses in seropositive dogs. J Am Vet Med Assoc 2002;220(1): 43–8.
34. Ellis JA, Gow SP, Lee LB, et al. Comparative efficacy of intranasal and injectable vaccines in stimulating *Bordetella bronchiseptica*-reactive anamnestic antibody responses in household dogs. Can Vet J 2017;58(8):809–15.
35. Griffin DE, Lin W-H, Pan C-H. Measles virus, immune control and persistence. FEMS Microbiol Rev 2012;36(3):649–62.
36. Beineke A, Puff C, Seehusen F, et al. Pathogenesis and immunopathology of systemic and nervous canine distemper. Vet Immunol Immunopathol 2009;127(1–2): 1–18.

37. Holzmann H, Hengel H, Tenbusch M. Eradication of measles: remaining challenges. Med Microbiol Immunol 2016;205:201–8.
38. Ellis JA, Gow SP, Mahan S, et al. Duration of immunity to experimental infection with bovine respiratory syncytial virus following intranasal vaccination of passively immune calves. J Am Vet Med Assoc 2013;243(11):1602–8.
39. Poorani R, Bhatt AN, Dwarakanath BS, et al. COX-2, aspirin and metabolism of arachidonic, eicosapentaenoic and docosahexaenic acids and their physiological and clinical significance. Eur J Pharmacol 2016;785:116–32.
40. Murphy JT, Sommer S, Kabara EA, et al. Gene expression profiling of monocyte-derived macrophages following infection with *Mycobacterium avium* subspecies *avium* and *Mycobacterium avium* subspecies *paratuberculosis*. Physiol Genomics 2006;28(1):67–75.
41. Wills RJ. Clinical pharmacokinetics of interferons. Clin Pharmacokinet 1990;19(5): 390–9.
42. Netea MG, Quintin J, van der Meer JWM. Trained immunity: a memory for innate host defense. Cell Host Microbe 2011;9:355–61.
43. Mackaness GB. The immunological basis of acquired cellular resistance. J Exp Med 1964;120:105–20.
44. Kurtz J, Franz K. Innate defence: evidence for memory in invertebrate immunity. Nature 2003;425:37–8.
45. Dangl JL, Jones JD. Plant pathogens and integrated defence responses to infection. Nature 2001;411:826–33.
46. Todd JD, Volenec FJ, Paton IM. Interferon in nasal secretions and sera of calves after intranasal administration of avirulent infectious bovine rhinotracheitis virus: association of interferon in nasal secretions with early resistance to challenge with virulent virus. Infect Immun 1972;5(5):699–706.
47. Bradley A, Kinyon J, Frana T, et al. Efficacy of intranasal administration of a modified live feline herpesvirus 1 and feline calicivirus vaccine against disease caused by Bordetella bronchiseptica after experimental challenge. J Vet Intern Med 2012;26(5):1121–5.
48. Blok BA, Arts RJW, Van Crevel R, et al. Trained innate immunity as underlying mechanism for the long-term, nonspecific effects of vaccines. J Leukoc Biol 2015;98(3):347–56.
49. Goodridge HS, Ahmed SS, Curtis N, et al. Harnessing the beneficial heterologous effects of vaccination. Nat Rev Immunol 2016;16(6):392–400.
50. Farber DL, Yudanin NA, Restifo NP. Human memory T cells: generation compartmentalization and homeostasis. Nat Rev Immunol 2014;14:24–35.
51. Capolunghi F, Rosado MM, Sinibaldi M, et al. Why do we need IgM memory B cells? Immunol Lett 2013;152:114–20.
52. Amanna IJ, Slifka MK. Mechanisms that determine plasma cell lifespan and duration of humoral immunity. Immunol Rev 2010;236:125–38.
53. Zinkernagel R. On plasma cell longevity or brevity. Expert Rev Vaccines 2014; 13(7):821–3.
54. Zinkernagel R, Hengartner H. Protective 'immunity' by pre-existing neutralizing antibody titers and preactivated T cells but not by so-called 'immunological memory'. Immunol Rev 2006;211:310–9.
55. Farber DL, Netea MG, Radbruch A, et al. Immunological memory: lessons from the past and a look to the future. Nat Rev Immunol 2016;16(2):124–8.
56. Campos M, Godson DL. The effectiveness and limitations of immune memory: understanding protective immune responses. Int J Parasitol 2003;33(5–6): 655–61.

57. Zinkernagel RM. Immunological memory protective immunity. Cell Mol Life Sci 2012;69(10):1635–40.
58. Coyne KP, Gaskell RM, Dawson S, et al. Evolutionary mechanisms of persistence and diversification of a calicivirus within endemically natural host populations. J Virol 2007;81(4):1961–71.
59. Pedersen NC, Hawkins KF. Mechanisms for persistence of acute and chronic feline calicivirus infections in the face of vaccination. Vet Microbiol 1995;47:141–56.
60. Giovanni G, Nicoletta V, Parvane K, et al. Prevention of herpes zoster and its complications: from clinic to real-life experience with the vaccine. J Med Microbiol 2016;65:1363–9.
61. Plotkin SA. Correlates of vaccine-induced immunity. Clin Infect Dis 2008;47:401–9.
62. Wadman M. The vaccine race: science, politics, and the human costs of defeating disease. New York: Viking; 2016.
63. Brown CM, Slavinski S, Ettestad P. Compendium of animal rabies prevention. J Am Vet Med Assoc 2016;248(5):505–17.
64. Rabies vaccine, killed virus. United States Department of Agriculture. 9 CFR 113.209.
65. Rabies vaccine, live virus. United States Department of Agriculture. 9 CFR 113.213.
66. Davis BM, Rall GF, Schnell MJ. Everything you always wanted to know about rabies virus (but were afraid to ask). Annu Rev Virol 2015;2:451–71.
67. Kennedy LJ, Lunt M, Barnes A. Factors influencing the antibody response of dogs vaccinated against rabies. Vaccine 2007;25:8500–7.
68. Gnanadurai CW, Zhou M, He W, et al. Presence of virus neutralizing antibodies in cerebral spinal fluid correlates with non-lethal rabies in dogs. PLoS Negl Trop Dis 2013;7(9):e2375.
69. Manning SE, Rupprecht CE, Fishbein D, et al. Human rabies prevention-United States 2008. Recommendations of the Advisory Committee on immunization practices. MMWR Recomm Rep 2008;57(RR-3):1–28.

Veterinary Oncology Immunotherapies

Philip J. Bergman, DVM, MS, PhD[a,b,c,*]

KEYWORDS

- Veterinary immunotherapy • Antibody-based therapy • Cancer vaccines

KEY POINTS

- The immune system is generally divided into 2 primary components: the innate immune response and the highly specific but more slowly developing adaptive or acquired immune response.
- Immune responses can be further separated by whether they are induced by exposure to a foreign antigen (an active response) or if they are transferred through serum or lymphocytes from an immunized individual (a passive response).
- The ideal cancer immunotherapy agent should be able to discriminate between cancer and normal cells (ie, specificity), be potent enough to kill small or large numbers of tumor cells (ie, sensitivity), and be able to prevent recurrence of the tumor (ie, durability).
- Tumor immunology and immunotherapy are among the most exciting and rapidly expanding fields; cancer immunotherapy is now recognized as a pillar of treatment alongside surgery, radiation, and chemotherapy.

The term immunity derived from the Latin word immunitas, which refers to the legal protection afforded to Roman senators holding office. Although the immune system is normally thought of as providing protection against infectious disease, the immune system's ability to recognize and eliminate cancer is the fundamental rationale for the immunotherapy of cancer. Multiple lines of evidence support a role for the immune system in managing cancer. These include (1) spontaneous remissions in patients with cancer without treatment; (2) the presence of tumor-specific cytotoxic T cells within tumor or draining lymph nodes; (3) the presence of monocytic, lymphocytic, and plasmacytic cellular infiltrates in tumors; (4) the increased incidence of some types of cancer in immunosuppressed patients; and (5) documentation of cancer remissions with the use of immunomodulators.[1,2] With the tools of molecular biology and a greater understanding of mechanisms to harness the immune system, effective tumor immunotherapy is now a reality. This new class of therapeutics offers a more targeted and,

The author discloses minor royalty stream for Oncept melanoma vaccine.
[a] Clinical Studies, VCA, Los Angeles, CA, USA; [b] Katonah Bedford Veterinary Center, Bedford Hills, NY, USA; [c] Memorial Sloan-Kettering Cancer Center, New York, NY, USA
* Katonah Bedford Veterinary Center, Bedford Hills, NY.
E-mail address: philip.bergman@vca.com

vetsmall.theclinics.com

therefore, more precise approach to the treatment of cancer. Cancer immunotherapy is now recognized as a pillar of treatment, alongside surgery, radiation, and chemotherapy.

TUMOR IMMUNOLOGY
Cellular Components

The immune system is generally divided into 2 primary components: the innate immune response and the highly specific but more slowly developing adaptive or acquired immune response. Innate immunity is rapid acting, although typically not very specific, and includes physicochemical barriers (eg, skin and mucosa); blood proteins, such as complement, phagocytic cells (macrophages, neutrophils, dendritic cells [DCs], and natural killer [NK] cells); and cytokines, which coordinate and regulate the cells involved in innate immunity. Adaptive immunity is thought of as the acquired arm of immunity that allows for exquisite specificity, an ability to remember the previous existence of the pathogen (ie, memory); differentiate self from nonself; and, importantly, the ability to respond more vigorously on repeat exposure to the pathogen. Adaptive immunity consists of T and B lymphocytes. The T cells are further divided into CD8 and major histocompatibility complex (MHC) class I cytotoxic helper T cells (CD4 and MHC class II), NK cells, and regulatory T (Treg) cells. B lymphocytes produce antibodies (Abs; humoral system), which may activate complement, enhance phagocytosis of opsonized target cells, and induce Ab-dependent cellular cytotoxicity. B-cell responses to tumors are thought by many investigators to be less important than the development of T-cell–mediated immunity; however, there is little evidence to fully support this notion.[3] The innate and adaptive arms of immunity are not mutually exclusive. They are linked by (1) the innate response's ability to stimulate and influence the nature of the adaptive response and (2) the sharing of effector mechanisms between innate and adaptive immune responses.

Immune responses can be further separated by whether they are induced by exposure to a foreign antigen (an active response) or if they are transferred through serum or lymphocytes from an immunized individual (a passive response). Although both approaches have the ability to be extremely specific for an antigen of interest, an important difference is the inability of passive approaches to generally confer memory. The principal components of the active or adaptive immune system are lymphocytes, antigen-presenting cells, and effector cells. Furthermore, responses can be subdivided by whether they are specific for a certain antigen or a nonspecific response whereby immunity is attempted to be conferred by upregulating the immune system without a specific target. These definitions are helpful because they allow methodologies to be more completely characterized, such as active-specific, passive-nonspecific, and so forth.

Immune Surveillance

The idea that the immune system may actively prevent the development of neoplasia is termed cancer immunosurveillance. Sound scientific evidence supports some aspects of this hypothesis,[4–7] including (1) interferon (IFN)-γ protects mice against the growth of tumors, (2) mice lacking IFN-γ receptor were more sensitive to chemically induced sarcomas than normal mice and were more likely to spontaneously develop tumors, (3) mice lacking major components of the adaptive immune response (T and B cells) have a high rate of spontaneous tumors, and (4) mice that lack IFN-γ and B or T cells develop tumors, especially at a young age.

Immune Evasion by Tumors

There are significant barriers to the generation of effective antitumor immunity by the host. Many tumors evade surveillance mechanisms and grow in immunocompetent hosts as easily illustrated by the overwhelming numbers of people and animals succumbing to cancer. There are multiple ways in which tumors evade the immune response, including (1) immunosuppressive cytokine production (eg, transforming growth factor (TGF)-β and interleukin [IL]-10)[8,9]; (2) impaired DC function via inactivation (anergy) and/or poor DC maturation through changes in IL-6/IL-10/vascular endothelial growth factor (VEGF)/granulocyte colony stimulating factor (GM-CSF)[10]; (3) induction of cells called Treg, which were initially called suppressor T cells (CD4/CD25/cytotoxic T lymphocyte associated (CTLA)-4/glucocorticoid-induced TNFR family related gene (GITR)/Foxp3 positive cells that can suppress tumor-specific CD4/CD8+ T cells)[11]; (4) MHC I loss through structural defects, changes in B2-microglobulin synthesis, defects in transporter-associated antigen processing, or actual MHC I gene loss (ie, allelic or locus loss); and (5) MHC I antigen presentation loss through B7-1 attenuation (B7-1 is an important costimulatory molecule for CD28-mediated T-cell receptor and MHC engagement) when the MHC system remains intact (see previous list item).

NONSPECIFIC TUMOR IMMUNOTHERAPY

Dr William Coley, a New York surgeon in the early 1900s, noted that some patients with cancer who developed incidental bacterial infections survived longer than those without infection.[12] Coley developed a bacterial vaccine (killed cultures of *Serratia marcescens* and *Streptococcus pyogenes* known as Coley toxins) to treat people with sarcomas that provided complete response rates of approximately 15%. Unfortunately, high failure rates and significant side effects lead to discontinuation of this approach. His seminal work laid the foundation for nonspecific modulation of the immune response in the treatment of cancer. There are numerous nonspecific tumor immunotherapy approaches, ranging from biological response modifiers (BRMs) to recombinant cytokines (see later discussion).

Biological Response Modifiers

BRMs are molecules that can modify the biological response of cells to changes in its external environment, which in the context of cancer immunotherapy could easily span nonspecific and specific immunotherapies. This section discusses nonspecific BRMs (sometimes termed immunopotentiators), which are often related to bacteria and/or viruses.

One of the earliest BRM discoveries after Coley toxin was the use of bacillus Calmette-Guérin (BCG; interestingly, Guérin was a veterinarian). BCG is the live attenuated strain of *Mycobacterium bovis* and intravesical instillation in the urinary bladder causes a significant local inflammatory response, which results in antitumor responses.[13] The use of BCG in veterinary patients was first reported by Owen and Bostock[14] in 1974 and has been investigated with numerous types of cancers, including urinary bladder carcinoma, osteosarcoma, lymphoma, prostatic carcinoma, transmissible venereal tumor, mammary tumors, sarcoids, squamous cell carcinoma, and others.[14–18] LDI-100, a product containing BCG and human chorionic gonadotropin, was compared with vinblastine in dogs with measurable grade II or III mast cell tumors.[19] Response rates were 28.6% and 11.7%, respectively, and the LDI-100 group had significantly less neutropenia. It is particularly exciting for veterinary cancer immunotherapy to potentially be able to use a BRM product, which has greater efficacy and less toxicity than a chemotherapy standard of care. Unfortunately, LDI-100 is not commercially available currently.

Corynebacterium parvum is another BRM that has been investigated for several tumors in veterinary medicine, including melanoma and mammary carcinoma.[20,21] Other bacterially derived BRMs include attenuated *Salmonella typhimurium* (VNP20009), mycobacterial cell wall DNA complexes (currently abstracts only), and bacterial superantigens.[22,23] Mycobacterial cell walls contain muramyl dipeptide (MDP), which can activate monocytes and tissue macrophages. MTP-PE (muramyl tripeptide-phosphatidylethanolamine) is an analog of MDP. When encapsulated in multilamellar liposomes (L-MTP-PE), monocytes and macrophages uptake MTP, leading to activation and subsequent tumoricidal effects through induction of multiple cytokines, including IL-1a, IL-1b, IL-7, IL-8, IL-12, and tumor necrosis factor.[24] L-MTP-PE has been investigated in numerous tumors in human and veterinary patients, including osteosarcoma, hemangiosarcoma, and mammary carcinoma.[24–28]

Oncolytic viruses have also been used as nonspecific anticancer BRMs in human and veterinary patients.[29] Adenoviruses have been engineered to transcriptionally target canine osteosarcoma cells and have been tested in vitro and in normal dogs with no major signs of virus-associated side effects.[30–32] Similarly, canine distemper virus (CDV), the canine equivalent of human measles virus, has been used in vitro to infect canine lymphocyte cell lines and neoplastic lymphocytes from dogs with B-cell and T-cell lymphoma,[33] with high infectivity rates, suggesting that CDV may be investigated in the future for treatment of dogs with lymphoma.

Imiquimod (Aldara) is a novel BRM that is a toll-like receptor 7 agonist.[34] Imiquimod has been reported as a successful treatment of Bowen disease (multicentric squamous cell carcinoma in situ) and other skin diseases in humans. Twelve cats with Bowen-like disease were treated topically with imiquimod 5% cream; initial and all subsequent new lesions responded in all cats.[35] An additional cat (with pinnal actinic keratoses and squamous cell carcinoma) and dog with cutaneous melanocytomas have subsequently been reported to have been successfully treated with topical imiquimod 5% cream.[36,37] Therefore, it seems that imiquimod 5% cream is well-tolerated, and further studies are warranted to further examine its usefulness in cats and dogs with other skin tumors that are not treatable through standardized means.

Recombinant Cytokines, Growth Factors, and Hormones

Several investigations using recombinant cytokines, growth factors, or hormones in various fashions for human and veterinary patients with cancer have been reported to date. Many have investigated the in vitro and/or in vivo effects of the soluble cytokine (eg, interferons, IL-2, IL-12, IL-15, and so forth with or without suicide gene therapy)[38–50]; liposome encapsulation of the cytokine (eg, liposomal IL-2)[39,51–54]; or use a virus, cell, liposome-DNA complex, plasmid, or other mechanism to expresses the cytokine (eg, recombinant poxvirus expressing IL-2).[51,55–62] Notably, the European Committee for Medicinal Products for Veterinary Use adopted a positive opinion in March, 2013, for the veterinary product Oncept IL-2 (feline pox virus expressing recombinant feline IL-2). This product also received conditional licensure from the US Department of Agriculture (USDA) Center for Veterinary Biologics (CVB) in 2015. It is labeled for use in addition to surgery and radiation in cats with stage I fibrosarcomas without metastasis or lymph node involvement, to reduce the risk of relapse and increase the time to relapse.

SPECIFIC TUMOR IMMUNOTHERAPY
Overview

The ultimate goal for a tumor immunotherapy with a specific target is elicitation of an antitumor immune response, which results in clinical regression of a tumor and/or its metastases. There are numerous types of specific tumor immunotherapies in phase I to III trials across a wide range of tumor types. Responses to cancer vaccines and other cancer immunotherapies may take several months or more to appear due to the slower speed of induction of the adaptive arm of the immune system as outlined in **Table 1**. This has necessitated the development of an alternative and more immunotherapeutic-based response system for human studies and this is highly likely necessary in the future for veterinary studies.[63] The ideal cancer immunotherapy agent would be able to discriminate between cancer and normal cells (ie, specificity), be potent enough to kill small or large numbers of tumor cells (ie, sensitivity), and be able to prevent recurrence of the tumor (ie, durability).

The immune system detects tumors through specific tumor-associated antigens (TAAs) and/or abnormal disease-associated antigens (DAAs) that are potentially recognized by both cytotoxic T lymphocytes and Abs.[64–66] TAAs and/or DAAs may be common to a particular tumor type, be unique to an individual tumor or may arise from mutated gene products such as ras, p53, p21, and/or others. Although unique TAAs may be more immunogenic than the other aforementioned shared tumor antigens, they are not practical targets because of their narrow specificity. Most shared tumor antigens are normal cellular antigens that are overexpressed in tumors. The first group to be identified was termed cancer testes antigens due to expression in normal testes; however, they are also found in melanoma and various other solid tumors, such as the MAGE/BAGE gene family. This article highlights those approaches that seem to hold particular promise in human clinical trials and many that have been tested to date in veterinary medicine.

To date, a variety of approaches has been taken to focus the immune system on the aforementioned targets. These include (1) whole cell, tumor cell lysate and/or subunit vaccines (autologous or made from a patient's own tumor tissue, allogeneic or made from individuals within a species bearing the same type of cancer, or whole cell vaccines from γ-irradiated tumor cell lines with or without immunostimulatory cytokines)[57,67–80]; (2) DNA vaccines that immunize with syngeneic and/or xenogeneic (different species than recipient) plasmid DNA designed to elicit antigen-specific humoral and cellular immunity[81–87] (see later discussion); (3) viral and/or viral vector-based methodologies designed to deliver genes encoding TAAs and/or immunostimulatory cytokines[88–93]; and (4) DC or CD40-activated B-cell vaccines (commonly loaded or transfected with TAAs, DNA or RNA from TAAs, or tumor lysates),[94–101] and adoptive cell transfer (the transfer of specific populations of immune effector cells to

Table 1
Comparison of chemotherapy and various antitumor immunotherapies

Treatment Type	Mechanism of Action	TAA or Target-Dependent	Specificity	Sensitivity	Response Time	Durability of Response
Chemotherapy	Cytotoxicity	No	Poor	Variable	Hours–days	Variable
Antitumor Vaccine	Immune Response	Yes	Good	Good	Weeks–months	Variable–long
Monoclonal Antibodies	Immune Response	Yes	Good	Good	Weeks	Variable
Checkpoint Inhibitors	Immune Response	No	Low	Moderate	Weeks–months	Long

Abbreviation: TAA, tumor-associated antigen.

generate a more powerful and focused antitumor immune response [see later discussion] with clinically relevant recent advances).[102]

Antibody-Based Therapies

Ab approaches for cancer immunotherapy include monoclonal Abs (mAbs)[103,104]; antiidiotype Abs (an idiotype is an immunoglobulin sequence unique to each B lymphocyte and therefore Abs directed against these idiotypes are referred to as antiidiotype)[105]; conjugated Abs (Ab conjugated to a toxin, chemotherapy, radionuclide, and so forth)[106]; and engineered Ab variants,[107,108] such as bispecific mAbs (can bind to 2 different targets at the same time), single-chain variable fragments (often used as artificial T-cell receptors), single-chain Abs, and so forth.

Rituximab (antihuman CD20 mAb; Rituxan, Biogen & Genentech, Inc [South San Francisco, CA]) was the first mAb approved by the US Food and Drug Administration (FDA)[109] in 1997 and, as of August 2017, there are more than 75 FDA-approved mAbs for the treatment of various human cancers. In those 20 years, a remarkably greater understanding of protein-engineering techniques and reciprocation between the immune system and cancer cells, as well as mechanisms of action and resistance for mAbs, have allowed for therapeutic Ab development to explode.[108,110]

Based on the significant improvement in remission and survival length of human patients with B-cell non-Hodgkin lymphoma (NHL) treated with rituximab and standard-of-care multiagent chemotherapy (and the lack of rituximab binding to canine CD20), numerous groups in veterinary medicine are in pursuit of similar caninized or felinized anti-CD20 mAb approaches.[111–117] Particular initial excitement and promise was noted in early pilot studies with caninized anti-CD20 and CD-52 mAbs (Vet Therapeutics, San Diego, CA; then purchased by Aratana, Inc) for canine B-cell and T-cell NHL, respectively. In 2015 and 2016, each product (Blontress and Tactress, respectively) received USDA-CVB licensure; however, subsequent unpublished studies did not show target binding or improvement in clinical outcomes compared with standard-of-care chemotherapy. Based on rituximab's remarkable track record and continually expanding list of indications (within the previously envisioned area of B-cell neoplasia but now outside of oncology in the treatment of nononcologic B-cell disorders), this author looks ardently forward to the clinical development of 1E4 (other anti-CD20 mAbs), as well as other mAb targets for dogs, cats, and other veterinary species afflicted with cancer and other diseases.[118–123]

Cancer Vaccines

One particularly exciting vaccine approach is the use of a HER-2 targeting attenuated listeria therapeutic vaccine.[124] This approach was used by Mason and colleagues[125] in dogs with appendicular osteosarcoma after being treated with amputation and adjuvant carboplatin chemotherapy. The results from this phase I study are particularly exciting because it translated into a median survival time approaching 3 years. It is currently unknown how much of the therapeutic efficacy is from the xenogeneic human HER-2 versus the listeria; however, in the future, it may be considered with other HER-2–related histologies. This product is currently undergoing further safety and efficacy studies by Aratana as AT-014 and it is anticipated this product will receive a USDA-CVB conditional license in late 2017 or early 2018.

This author has developed a xenogeneic DNA vaccine program for melanoma in collaboration with human investigators from Memorial Sloan-Kettering Cancer Center.[126,127] Preclinical and clinical studies by our laboratory and others have shown that xenogeneic DNA vaccination with tyrosinase family members (eg, tyrosinase, GP100, GP75) can produce immune responses resulting in tumor rejection or protection and prolongation of survival, whereas syngeneic vaccination with orthologous DNA does not induce immune responses. Although tyrosinase may not seem to be a preferred target in amelanotic canine melanoma owing to poor expression when assessed by immunohistochemistry,[128] more appropriate or sensitive PCR-based studies and other immunohistochemistry-based studies document significant tyrosinase overexpression in melanotic and amelanotic melanomas across species.[129–134] These studies provided the impetus for development of a xenogeneic tyrosinase (or similar melanosomal glycoproteins) DNA vaccine program in canine malignant melanoma (CMM). Cohorts of dogs received increasing doses of xenogeneic plasmid DNA encoding human tyrosinase (huTyr), murine GP75, murine tyrosinase (muTyr), muTyr plus or minus HuGM-CSF (both administered as plasmid DNA), or muTyr off-study intramuscularly biweekly for a total of 4 vaccinations. The author and collaborators have investigated the Ab and T-cell responses in dogs vaccinated with huTyr. Antigen-specific (huTyr) IFN-γ T cells were found along with 2-fold to 5-fold increases in circulating Abs to huTyr, which can cross-react to canine tyrosinase, suggesting the breaking of tolerance.[135,136] Clinical results with prolongation in survival have been reported.[126,127] The results of these trials demonstrate that xenogeneic DNA vaccination in CMM (1) is safe; (2) leads to the development of antityrosinase Abs and T cells; (3) is potentially therapeutic; and (4) is an attractive candidate for further evaluation in an adjuvant, minimal residual disease, phase II setting for CMM. Based on these studies, a multiinstitutional safety and efficacy trial for USDA licensure in dogs with locally controlled stage II to III oral melanoma was initiated in 2006 with granting of conditional licensure in 2007, which represented the first US governmental regulatory agency approval of a vaccine to treat cancer across species. Results of this licensure trial documented a statistically significant improvement in survival for vaccinates versus controls and a full licensure for the huTyr-based canine melanoma vaccine from USDA-CVB was received in December 2009 (Oncept, Merial, Inc [Boerhinger Animal Health, Duluth, GA]).[137]

Herzog and colleagues[138] studied concurrent use of Oncept and external beam radiation because many dogs with oral malignant melanoma may not be able to undergo surgery for local tumor control. This pilot study determined that concurrent use was well-tolerated with no unexpected toxicities. Ottnod and colleagues[139] performed a single-site retrospective study on 30 dogs with stage II to III oral malignant melanoma (15 each with and without use of Oncept). They determined that those dogs receiving Oncept did not achieve a greater progression-free survival, disease-free interval, or median survival time than dogs that did not receive the vaccine. Contrary to the aforementioned prospective USDA 5-site licensure trial,[137] this study had less than 35% of cases treated surgically with margins 1 mm or more, suggesting a significant lack of local tumor control. Furthermore, contrary to the aforementioned prospective USDA 5-site licensure trial, the Ottnod and colleagues[139–143] study, similar to other noncontrolled retrospective studies, either had a wide variety of other treatments used in both the nonvaccinated and vaccinated groups, had small numbers of patients investigated, and/or the cause (in the context of local or distant disease) of death and/or progression of disease was not reported. At the 2016 Veterinary Cancer Society meeting, this author reported the outcomes of 320 dogs with malignant melanoma treated with Oncept across VCA oncology centers. The long-term median outcomes noted in that study are extremely similar to those we reported from the USDA 5-site prospective licensure trial and compare highly favorably to outcomes reported with standardized therapies without Oncept. Not surprisingly, the smaller poorly controlled retrospective studies do not seem to mirror the results seen in larger and more highly controlled studies.

Human clinical trials using various xenogeneic melanosomal antigens as DNA (or peptide with adjuvant) vaccination began in 2005 and the preliminary results look favorable.[144–146] To further highlight xenogeneic DNA vaccination as a platform to target other possible antigens for other histologies, we have completed a phase I trial of murine CD20 for dogs with B-cell lymphoma (USDA-CVB conditionally licensed as Canine Lymphoma Vaccine from Merial, Inc and currently undergoing further efficacy studies in larger numbers of dogs) and we have also investigated the efficacy of local tumor control and use of xenogeneic DNA vaccination in dogs with digit malignant melanoma.[147] These investigations led to the development of a canine digit melanoma staging scheme and found an improvement in survival compared with historical outcomes with digit amputation only. The author has also documented a decreased prognosis for dogs with advanced stage disease and/or increased time from digit amputation to the start of vaccination. Phillips and colleagues[129,148] have also reported the overexpression of tyrosinase in equine melanoma, determined the safety and optimal use of the needle-free delivery device into the pectoral region with Oncept, and documented antigen-specific humoral responses after vaccination in all horses. Oncept also seems to be safe for use in cats.[149]

A small subset of dogs with malignant melanoma have exon 11 KIT gene mutations[150,151]; therefore, the more routine use of KIT testing by PCR of CMM and subsequent use of c-kit small molecule inhibitors (particularly in dogs with advanced stage disease and/or lack of response to Oncept) should be considered. Furthermore, with somatic mutations in NRAS and PTEN being found in CMM,[152] similar to human melanoma hotspot sites, these may represent logical druggable targets in the future.

THE FUTURE OF CANCER IMMUNOTHERAPY

Tumor immunology and immunotherapy is currently among the most exciting and rapidly expanding fields. Significant resources are focused on mechanisms to simultaneously maximally stimulate an antitumor immune response while minimizing the immunosuppressive aspects of the tumor microenvironment.[8] The recent elucidation and blockade of immunosuppressive cytokines (eg, TGF-β, IL-10, and IL-13) and/or the negative costimulatory molecule CTLA-4[153,154] and PD-1 (Programmed Cell Death 1 or CD279),[155] along with the functional characterization of myeloid-derived suppressor cells and Treg cells,[156–159] have dramatically improved cell-mediated immunity to tumors by taking the brake off the immune system. Immunotherapy is unlikely to become a sole modality in the treatment of cancer because the traditional modalities of surgery, radiation, and/or chemotherapy are extremely likely to be used in combination with immunotherapy in the future. Like any form of anticancer treatment, immunotherapy seems to work best in a minimal residual disease setting, suggesting its most appropriate use will be in an adjuvant setting with local tumor therapies such as surgery and/or radiation.[160] Similarly, the long-held belief that chemotherapy (noncorticosteroid) attenuates immune responses from cancer vaccines is beginning to be disproven through investigations on a variety of levels.[161,162]

The aforementioned greatly expanded understanding of the molecular immune system has recently translated into human cancer immunotherapeutics that confer a survival benefit, such as the use of the checkpoint inhibitor anti-CTLA-4 Ab, ipilimumab (Yervoy, Bristol-Myers Squibb [New York, NY]); and the selective BRAF inhibitors, vemurafenib (Zelboraf, Genentech) and dabrafenib (GSK2118436, GlaxoSmithKline [Brentford, Middlesex, United Kingdom]), in patients who are BRAF V600-mutation–positive. Currently, FDA-approved Abs directed against another checkpoint inhibitor, known as PD-1 receptor, or against human PDL-1 (L, ligand), such as nivolumab

(Opdivo, Bristol-Myers Squibb) and pembrolizumab (Keytruda, Merck [Kenilworth, NJ]), have generated the most excitement due to approximately 20% to 30% of human patients having durable objective tumor responses.[155,163] The highest objective tumor response rates have been seen to date in patients treated with concurrent PD-1 and CTLA-4 checkpoint inhibitors.[155,164,165] Furthermore, pembrolizumab was recently given FDA approval for unresectable or metastatic, microsatellite instability-high (MSI-H) or mismatch repair deficient (dMMR) solid tumors that have progressed following prior treatment.[166] This is truly revolutionary because it represents the first cancer-agnostic FDA approval and is among many recent FDA approvals based on single-arm studies. There are currently more than 100 different checkpoint inhibitors in development and the immunooncology (IO) pendulum has swung from the previous primarily target-dependent approaches to the current checkpoint inhibitor target-independent approach. The IO pendulum over time is likely to come back to the middle with a concurrent target-dependent approach (ie, vaccine or similar) alongside target-independent checkpoint inhibitors.[167,168]

Unfortunately, very few biomarkers of response with these clinically important agents have been found to date except for tumors that generate numerous neoantigens from tumor-specific mutations.[169,170] This further highlights why pembrolizumab was given FDA approval for MSI-H or dMMR solid tumors because these tumors throw off comparatively much higher numbers of neoantigens. A new and highly innovative personalized human cancer vaccine that takes advantage of this biomarker-based approach uses the neoantigens specific to that individual's cancer because they are not present in normal tissues and are highly immunogenic.[171]

Another area of extreme promise in IO is a form of adoptive cell therapy called chimeric antigen receptor (CAR)-T cells. T cells are harvested from a patient and then genetically engineered to express a CAR on their cell surface with expansion in vitro before being reinfused back into the patient.[172] This CAR is specifically designed to recognize a specific TAA with a domain responsible for activating the T cell when the CAR-T binds its TAA. The latest generations of CAR-T are engineered to contain important costimulatory domains that further enhance the immune response against the cancer cell containing the TAA. On July 12, 2017, an expert panel of the FDA, the Oncologic Drugs Advisory Committee, unanimously (10 to 0) recommended approval of CTL019 (tisagenlecleucel), an investigational CAR-T therapy using CD19 as its CAR of choice for patients with B-cell acute lymphoblastic leukemia. Many CAR-T studies have found greater than 80% to 90% objective tumor responses; however, side effects, including death, can occur.[172] Furthermore, CAR-Ts are currently difficult to make and carry a high cost of goods to produce, making for a difficult but not impossible commercial development path in veterinary medicine.

Checkpoints, checkpoint inhibitors, and other adoptive cell transfer technologies, such as CAR-T and others, are also starting to be better understood and pursued in veterinary diseases.[102,173–186] Furthermore, the exciting race to develop commercial veterinary specific IO therapeutics, such as checkpoint inhibitors and CAR-T, is currently ongoing with a handful of animal health companies. Because these therapeutics reduce immune tolerance and more easily generate specific antitumor immune responses in patients, pathologic autoimmunity was predicted and is now being seen clinically in human patients as a side effect.[164,187,188]

SUMMARY

The future looks extremely bright for immunotherapy. Similarly, the veterinary oncology profession is uniquely able to greatly contribute to the many advances to come. Unfortunately, what works in a mouse will often not reflect the outcome in human patients with cancer. Therefore, comparative immunotherapy studies using veterinary patients may be able to better bridge murine and human studies. To this end, a large number of cancers in dogs and cats seem to be remarkably stronger models for counterpart human tumors than presently available murine model systems.[152,189–196] This is likely due to a variety of reasons, including but not limited to extreme similarities in the biology of the tumors (eg, chemoresistance, radioresistance, sharing metastatic phenotypes, site selectivity), spontaneous syngeneic cancer (vs typically an induced and/or xenogeneic cancer in murine models), and, finally, that the dogs and cats that are spontaneously developing these tumors are outbred, immune-competent, and live in the same environment that humans do. This author ardently looks forward to the time when cancer immunotherapy plays the same significant role in the treatment and/or prevention of cancers in veterinary patients as it currently does in human cancers.

REFERENCES

1. Bergman PJ. Biologic response modification. In: Rosenthal RC, editor. Veterinary oncology secrets. 1st edition. Philadelphia: Hanley & Belfus, Inc.; 2001. p. 79–82.
2. Baxevanis CN, Perez SA, Papamichail M. Cancer immunotherapy. Crit Rev Clin Lab Sci 2009;46:167–89.
3. Reilly RT, Emens LA, Jaffee EM. Humoral and cellular immune responses: independent forces or collaborators in the fight against cancer? Curr Opin Investig Drugs 2001;2(1):133–5.
4. Smyth MJ, Godfrey DI, Trapani JA. A fresh look at tumor immunosurveillance and immunotherapy. Nat Immunol 2001;2(4):293–9.
5. Wallace ME, Smyth MJ. The role of natural killer cells in tumor control–effectors and regulators of adaptive immunity. Springer Semin Immunopathol 2005;27(1): 49–64.
6. Itoh H, Horiuchi Y, Nagasaki T, et al. Evaluation of immunological status in tumor-bearing dogs. Vet Immunol Immunopathol 2009;132(2–4):85–90.
7. Schmiedt CW, Grimes JA, Holzman G, et al. Incidence and risk factors for development of malignant neoplasia after feline renal transplantation and cyclosporine-based immunosuppression. Vet Comp Oncol 2009;7:45–53.
8. Catchpole B, Gould SM, Kellett-Gregory LM, et al. Immunosuppressive cytokines in the regional lymph node of a dog suffering from oral malignant melanoma. J Small Anim Pract 2002;43(10):464–7.
9. Zagury D, Gallo RC. Anti-cytokine Ab immune therapy: present status and perspectives. Drug Discov Today 2004;9(2):72–81.
10. Morse MA, Mosca PJ, Clay TM, et al. Dendritic cell maturation in active immunotherapy strategies. Expert Opin Biol Ther 2002;2(1):35–43.
11. Yamaguchi T, Sakaguchi S. Regulatory T cells in immune surveillance and treatment of cancer. Semin Cancer Biol 2006;16(2):115–23.
12. Richardson MA, Ramirez T, Russell NC, et al. Coley toxins immunotherapy: a retrospective review. Altern Ther Health Med 1999;5(3):42–7.
13. Herr HW, Morales A. History of bacillus Calmette-Guerin and bladder cancer: an immunotherapy success story. J Urol 2008;179:53–6.
14. Owen LN, Bostock DE. Proceedings: tumour therapy in dogs using B.C.G. Br J Cancer 1974;29:95.

15. MacEwen EG. An immunologic approach to the treatment of cancer. Vet Clin North Am 1977;7:65–75.

16. Theilen GH, Hills D. Comparative aspects of cancer immunotherapy: immunologic methods used for treatment of spontaneous cancer in animals. J Am Vet Med Assoc 1982;181:1134–41.

17. MacEwen EG. Approaches to cancer therapy using biological response modifiers. Vet Clin North Am Small Anim Pract 1985;15:667–88.

18. Klein WR, Rutten VP, Steerenberg PA, et al. The present status of BCG treatment in the veterinary practice. In Vivo 1991;5:605–8.

19. Henry CJ, Downing S, Rosenthal RC, et al. Evaluation of a novel immunomodulator composed of human chorionic gonadotropin and bacillus Calmette-Guerin for treatment of canine mast cell tumors in clinically affected dogs. Am J Vet Res 2007;68:1246–51.

20. Parodi AL, Misdorp W, Mialot JP, et al. Intratumoral BCG and *Corynebacterium parvum* therapy of canine mammary tumours before radical mastectomy. Cancer Immunol Immunother 1983;15:172–7.

21. MacEwen EG, Patnaik AK, Harvey HJ, et al. Canine oral melanoma: comparison of surgery versus surgery plus *Corynebacterium parvum*. Cancer Invest 1986; 4(5):397–402.

22. Thamm DH, Kurzman ID, King I, et al. Systemic administration of an attenuated, tumor-targeting *Salmonella typhimurium* to dogs with spontaneous neoplasia: phase I evaluation. Clin Cancer Res 2005;11:4827–34.

23. Dow SW, Elmslie RE, Willson AP, et al. In vivo tumor transfection with superantigen plus cytokine genes induces tumor regression and prolongs survival in dogs with malignant melanoma. J Clin Invest 1998;101:2406–14.

24. Kleinerman ES, Jia S-F, Griffin J, et al. Phase II study of liposomal muramyl tripeptide in osteosarcoma: The cytokine cascade and monocyte activation following administration. J Clin Oncol 1992;10:1310–6.

25. MacEwen EG, Kurzman ID, Vail DM, et al. Adjuvant therapy for melanoma in dogs: results of randomized clinical trials using surgery, liposome-encapsulated muramyl tripeptide, and granulocyte macrophage colony-stimulating factor. Clin Cancer Res 1999;5:4249–58.

26. Teske E, Rutteman GR, vd Ingh TS, et al. Liposome-encapsulated muramyl tripeptide phosphatidylethanolamine (L-MTP-PE): a randomized clinical trial in dogs with mammary carcinoma. Anticancer Res 1998;18:1015–9.

27. Kurzman ID, MacEwen EG, Rosenthal RC, et al. Adjuvant therapy for osteosarcoma in dogs: results of randomized clinical trials using combined liposome-encapsulated muramyl tripeptide and cisplatin. Clin Cancer Res 1995;1: 1595–601.

28. Vail DM, MacEwen EG, Kurzman ID, et al. Liposome-encapsulated muramyl tripeptide phosphatidylethanolamine adjuvant immunotherapy for splenic hemangiosarcoma in the dog: a randomized multi-institutional clinical trial. Clin Cancer Res 1995;1:1165–70.

29. Arendt M, Nasir L, Morgan IM. Oncolytic gene therapy for canine cancers: teaching old dog viruses new tricks. Vet Comp Oncol 2009;7:153–61.

30. Smith BF, Curiel DT, Ternovoi VV, et al. Administration of a conditionally replicative oncolytic canine adenovirus in normal dogs. Cancer Biother Radiopharm 2006;21:601–6.

31. Le LP, Rivera AA, Glasgow JN, et al. Infectivity enhancement for adenoviral transduction of canine osteosarcoma cells. Gene Ther 2006;13:389–99.

32. Hemminki A, Kanerva A, Kremer EJ, et al. A canine conditionally replicating adenovirus for evaluating oncolytic virotherapy in a syngeneic animal model. Mol Ther 2003;7:163–73.

33. Suter SE, Chein MB, von M, et al. In vitro canine distemper virus infection of canine lymphoid cells: a prelude to oncolytic therapy for lymphoma. Clin Cancer Res 2005;11:1579–87.

34. Meyer T, Stockfleth E. Clinical investigations of Toll-like receptor agonists. Expert Opin Investig Drugs 2008;17:1051–65.

35. Gill VL, Bergman PJ, Baer KE, et al. Use of imiquimod 5% cream (AldaraTM) in cats with multicentric squamous cell carcinoma in situ: 12 cases (2002-2005). Vet Comp Oncol 2008;6:55–64.

36. Peters-Kennedy J, Scott DW, Miller WH Jr. Apparent clinical resolution of pinnal actinic keratoses and squamous cell carcinoma in a cat using topical imiquimod 5% cream. J Feline Med Surg 2008;10(6):593–9.

37. Coyner K, Loeffler D. Topical imiquimod in the treatment of two cutaneous melanocytomas in a dog. Vet Dermatol 2012;23(2):145–9, e31.

38. Tateyama S, Priosoeryanto BP, Yamaguchi R, et al. In vitro growth inhibition activities of recombinant feline interferon on all lines derived from canine tumors. Res Vet Sci 1995;59:275–7.

39. Kruth SA. Biological response modifiers: interferons, interleukins, recombinant products, liposomal products. Vet Clin North Am Small Anim Pract 1998;28: 269–95.

40. Whitley EM, Bird AC, Zucker KE, et al. Modulation by canine interferon-gamma of major histocompatibility complex and tumor-associated antigen expression in canine mammary tumor and melanoma cell lines. Anticancer Res 1995;15: 923–9.

41. Hampel V, Schwarz B, Kempf C, et al. Adjuvant immunotherapy of feline fibrosarcoma with recombinant feline interferon-omega. J Vet Intern Med 2007;21: 1340–6.

42. Finocchiaro LM, Glikin GC. Cytokine-enhanced vaccine and suicide gene therapy as surgery adjuvant treatments for spontaneous canine melanoma. Gene Ther 2008;15:267–76.

43. Cutrera J, Torrero M, Shiomitsu K, et al. Intratumoral bleomycin and IL-12 electrochemogenetherapy for treating head and neck tumors in dogs. Methods Mol Biol 2008;423:319–25.

44. Finocchiaro LM, Fiszman GL, Karara AL, et al. Suicide gene and cytokines combined nonviral gene therapy for spontaneous canine melanoma. Cancer Gene Ther 2008;15:165–72.

45. Akhtar N, Padilla ML, Dickerson EB, et al. Interleukin-12 inhibits tumor growth in a novel angiogenesis canine hemangiosarcoma xenograft model. Neoplasia 2004;6:106–16.

46. Dickerson EB, Fosmire S, Padilla ML, et al. Potential to target dysregulated interleukin-2 receptor expression in canine lymphoid and hematopoietic malignancies as a model for human cancer. J Immunother 2002;25:36–45.

47. Okano F, Yamada K. Canine interleukin-18 induces apoptosis and enhances Fas ligand mRNA expression in a canine carcinoma cell line. Anticancer Res 2000; 20:3411–5.

48. Jahnke A, Hirschberger J, Fischer C, et al. Intra-tumoral gene delivery of feIL-2, feIFN-gamma and feGM-CSF using magnetofection as a neoadjuvant treatment option for feline fibrosarcomas: a phase-I study. J Vet Med A Physiol Pathol Clin Med 2007;54:599–606.

49. Dickerson EB, Akhtar N, Steinberg H, et al. Enhancement of the antiangiogenic activity of interleukin-12 by peptide targeted delivery of the cytokine to alphav-beta3 integrin. Mol Cancer Res 2004;2:663–73.

50. Finocchiaro LM, Fondello C, Gil-Cardeza ML, et al. Cytokine-enhanced vaccine and interferon-beta plus suicide gene therapy as surgery adjuvant treatments for spontaneous canine melanoma. Hum Gene Ther 2015;26:367–76.

51. Dow S, Elmslie R, Kurzman I, et al. Phase I study of liposome-DNA complexes encoding the interleukin-2 gene in dogs with osteosarcoma lung metastases. Hum Gene Ther 2005;16:937–46.

52. Skubitz KM, Anderson PM. Inhalational interleukin-2 liposomes for pulmonary metastases: a phase I clinical trial. Anticancer Drugs 2000;11:555–63.

53. Khanna C, Anderson PM, Hasz DE, et al. Interleukin-2 liposome inhalation therapy is safe and effective for dogs with spontaneous pulmonary metastases. Cancer 1997;79:1409–21.

54. Khanna C, Hasz DE, Klausner JS, et al. Aerosol delivery of interleukin 2 liposomes is nontoxic and biologically effective: canine studies. Clin Cancer Res 1996;2:721–34.

55. Jourdier TM, Moste C, Bonnet MC, et al. Local immunotherapy of spontaneous feline fibrosarcomas using recombinant poxviruses expressing interleukin 2 (IL2). Gene Ther 2003;10(26):2126–32.

56. Siddiqui F, Li CY, Zhang X, et al. Characterization of a recombinant adenovirus vector encoding heat-inducible feline interleukin-12 for use in hyperthermia-induced gene-therapy. Int J Hyperthermia 2006;22:117–34.

57. Quintin-Colonna F, Devauchelle P, Fradelizi D, et al. Gene therapy of spontaneous canine melanoma and feline fibrosarcoma by intratumoral administration of histoincompatible cells expressing human interleukin-2. Gene Ther 1996;3(12):1104–12.

58. Kamstock D, Guth A, Elmslie R, et al. Liposome-DNA complexes infused intravenously inhibit tumor angiogenesis and elicit antitumor activity in dogs with soft tissue sarcoma. Cancer Gene Ther 2006;13:306–17.

59. Junco JA, Basalto R, Fuentes F, et al. Gonadotrophin releasing hormone-based vaccine, an effective candidate for prostate cancer and other hormone-sensitive neoplasms. Adv Exp Med Biol 2008;617:581–7.

60. Chou PC, Chuang TF, Jan TR, et al. Effects of immunotherapy of IL-6 and IL-15 plasmids on transmissible venereal tumor in beagles. Vet Immunol Immunopathol 2009;130(1–2):25–34.

61. Chuang TF, Lee SC, Liao KW, et al. Electroporation-mediated IL-12 gene therapy in a transplantable canine cancer model. Int J Cancer 2009;125(3):698–707.

62. Finocchiaro LM, Glikin GC. Cytokine-enhanced vaccine and suicide gene therapy as surgery adjuvant treatments for spontaneous canine melanoma: 9 years of follow-up. Cancer Gene Ther 2012;19(12):852–61.

63. Seymour L, Bogaerts J, Perrone A, et al. iRECIST: guidelines for response criteria for use in trials testing immunotherapeutics. Lancet Oncol 2017;18:e143–52.

64. Bergman PJ. Anticancer vaccines. Vet Clin North Am Small Anim Pract 2007;37:1111–9.

65. Beatty PL, Finn OJ. Preventing cancer by targeting abnormally expressed self-antigens: MUC1 vaccines for prevention of epithelial adenocarcinomas. Ann N Y Acad Sci 2013;1284:52–6.

66. Regan D, Guth A, Coy J, et al. Cancer immunotherapy in veterinary medicine: current options and new developments. Vet J 2016;207:20–8.

67. Hogge GS, Burkholder JK, Culp J, et al. Preclinical development of human granulocyte-macrophage colony-stimulating factor-transfected melanoma cell vaccine using established canine cell lines and normal dogs. Cancer Gene Ther 1999;6(1):26–36.

68. Alexander AN, Huelsmeyer MK, Mitzey A, et al. Development of an allogeneic whole-cell tumor vaccine expressing xenogeneic gp100 and its implementation in a phase II clinical trial in canine patients with malignant melanoma. Cancer Immunol Immunother 2006;55(4):433–42.

69. U'Ren LW, Biller BJ, Elmslie RE, et al. Evaluation of a novel tumor vaccine in dogs with hemangiosarcoma. J Vet Intern Med 2007;21:113–20.

70. Bird RC, Deinnocentes P, Lenz S, et al. An allogeneic hybrid-cell fusion vaccine against canine mammary cancer. Vet Immunol Immunopathol 2008;123: 289–304.

71. Turek MM, Thamm DH, Mitzey A, et al. Human granulocyte & macrophage colony-stimulating factor DNA cationic-lipid complexed autologous tumour cell vaccination in the treatment of canine B-cell multicentric lymphoma. Vet Comp Oncol 2007;5:219–31.

72. Kuntsi-Vaattovaara H, Verstraete FJM, Newsome JT, et al. Resolution of persistent oral papillomatosis in a dog after treatment with a recombinant canine oral papillomavirus vaccine. Vet Comp Oncol 2003;1:57–63.

73. Milner RJ, Salute M, Crawford C, et al. The immune response to disialoganglioside GD3 vaccination in normal dogs: a melanoma surface antigen vaccine. Vet Immunol Immunopathol 2006;114:273–84.

74. Marconato L, Frayssinet P, Rouquet N, et al. Randomized, placebo-controlled, double-blinded chemo-immunotherapy clinical trial in a pet dog model of diffuse large B-cell lymphoma. Clin Cancer Res 2014;20(3):668–77.

75. Suckow MA. Cancer vaccines: harnessing the potential of anti-tumor immunity. Vet J 2013;198(1):28–33.

76. Epple LM, Bemis LT, Cavanaugh RP, et al. Prolonged remission of advanced bronchoalveolar adenocarcinoma in a dog treated with autologous, tumour-derived chaperone-rich cell lysate (CRCL) vaccine. Int J Hyperthermia 2013; 29(5):390–8.

77. Andersen BM, Pluhar GE, Seiler CE, et al. Vaccination for invasive canine meningioma induces in situ production of antibodies capable of antibody-dependent cell-mediated cytotoxicity. Cancer Res 2013;73(10):2987–97.

78. Yannelli JR, Wouda R, Masterson TJ, et al. Development of an autologous canine cancer vaccine system for resectable malignant tumors in dogs. Vet Immunol Immunopathol 2016;182:95–100.

79. Marconato L, Stefanello D, Sabattini S, et al. Enhanced therapeutic effect of APAVAC immunotherapy in combination with dose-intense chemotherapy in dogs with advanced indolent B-cell lymphoma. Vaccine 2015;33:5080–6.

80. Weir C, Hudson AL, Moon E, et al. Streptavidin: a novel immunostimulant for the selection and delivery of autologous and syngeneic tumor vaccines. Cancer Immunol Res 2014;2:469–79.

81. Kamstock D, Elmslie R, Thamm D, et al. Evaluation of a xenogeneic VEGF vaccine in dogs with soft tissue sarcoma. Cancer Immunol Immunother 2007;56: 1299–309.

82. Yu WY, Chuang TF, Guichard C, et al. Chicken HSP70 DNA vaccine inhibits tumor growth in a canine cancer model. Vaccine 2011;29(18):3489–500.

83. Impellizeri JA, Ciliberto G, Aurisicchio L. Electro-gene-transfer as a new tool for cancer immunotherapy in animals. Vet Comp Oncol 2014;12(4):310–8.
84. Denies S, Cicchelero L, Polis I, et al. Immunogenicity and safety of xenogeneic vascular endothelial growth factor receptor-2 DNA vaccination in mice and dogs. Oncotarget 2016;7:10905–16.
85. Gabai V, Venanzi FM, Bagashova E, et al. Pilot study of p62 DNA vaccine in dogs with mammary tumors. Oncotarget 2014;5:12803–10.
86. Riccardo F, Iussich S, Maniscalco L, et al. CSPG4-specific immunity and survival prolongation in dogs with oral malignant melanoma immunized with human CSPG4 DNA. Clin Cancer Res 2014;20:3753–62.
87. Gibson HM, Veenstra JJ, Jones R, et al. Induction of HER2 immunity in outbred domestic cats by DNA electrovaccination. Cancer Immunol Res 2015;3:777–86.
88. von EH, Sadeghi A, Carlsson B, et al. Efficient adenovector CD40 ligand immunotherapy of canine malignant melanoma. J Immunother 2008;31:377–84.
89. Johnston KB, Monteiro JM, Schultz LD, et al. Protection of beagle dogs from mucosal challenge with canine oral papillomavirus by immunization with recombinant adenoviruses expressing codon-optimized early genes. Virology 2005; 336:208–18.
90. Thacker EE, Nakayama M, Smith BF, et al. A genetically engineered adenovirus vector targeted to CD40 mediates transduction of canine dendritic cells and promotes antigen-specific immune responses in vivo. Vaccine 2009;27(50): 7116–24.
91. Peruzzi D, Mesiti G, Ciliberto G, et al. Telomerase and HER-2/neu as targets of genetic cancer vaccines in dogs. Vaccine 2010;28(5):1201–8.
92. Gavazza A, Lubas G, Fridman A, et al. Safety and efficacy of a genetic vaccine targeting telomerase plus chemotherapy for the therapy of canine B-cell lymphoma. Hum Gene Ther 2013;24(8):728–38.
93. Autio KP, Ruotsalainen JJ, Anttila MO, et al. Attenuated semliki forest virus for cancer treatment in dogs: safety assessment in two laboratory beagles. BMC Vet Res 2015;11:170.
94. Gyorffy S, Rodriguez-Lecompte JC, Woods JP, et al. Bone marrow-derived dendritic cell vaccination of dogs with naturally occurring melanoma by using human gp100 antigen. J Vet Intern Med 2005;19(1):56–63.
95. Tamura K, Arai H, Ueno E, et al. Comparison of dendritic cell-mediated immune responses among canine malignant cells. J Vet Med Sci 2007;69:925–30.
96. Tamura K, Yamada M, Isotani M, et al. Induction of dendritic cell-mediated immune responses against canine malignant melanoma cells. Vet J 2008;175: 126–9.
97. Rodriguez-Lecompte JC, Kruth S, Gyorffy S, et al. Cell-based cancer gene therapy: breaking tolerance or inducing autoimmunity? Anim Health Res Rev 2004; 5:227–34.
98. Kyte JA, Mu L, Aamdal S, et al. Phase I/II trial of melanoma therapy with dendritic cells transfected with autologous tumor-mRNA. Cancer Gene Ther 2006; 13:905–18.
99. Mason NJ, Coughlin CM, Overley B, et al. RNA-loaded CD40-activated B cells stimulate antigen-specific T-cell responses in dogs with spontaneous lymphoma. Gene Ther 2008;15:955–65.
100. Sorenmo KU, Krick E, Coughlin CM, et al. CD40-activated B cell cancer vaccine improves second clinical remission and survival in privately owned dogs with non-Hodgkin's lymphoma. PLoS One 2011;6(8):e24167.

101. Bird RC, Deinnocentes P, Church Bird AE, et al. An autologous dendritic cell canine mammary tumor hybrid-cell fusion vaccine. Cancer Immunol Immunother 2011;60(1):87–97.

102. O'Connor CM, Sheppard S, Hartline CA, et al. Adoptive T-cell therapy improves treatment of canine non-Hodgkin lymphoma post chemotherapy. Sci Rep 2012; 2:249.

103. Sharma P, Wagner K, Wolchok JD, et al. Novel cancer immunotherapy agents with survival benefit: recent successes and next steps. Nat Rev Cancer 2011; 11:805–12.

104. Singh S, Kumar N, Dwiwedi P, et al. Monoclonal antibodies: a review. Curr Clin Pharmacol 2017. [Epub ahead of print].

105. Ladjemi MZ. Anti-idiotypic antibodies as cancer vaccines: achievements and future improvements. Front Oncol 2012;2:158.

106. Thomas A, Teicher BA, Hassan R. Antibody-drug conjugates for cancer therapy. Lancet Oncol 2016;17:e254–62.

107. Ross SL, Sherman M, McElroy PL, et al. Bispecific T cell engager (BiTE®) antibody constructs can mediate bystander tumor cell killing. PLoS One 2017;12: e0183390.

108. Strohl WR. Current progress in innovative engineered antibodies. Protein Cell 2017. [Epub ahead of print].

109. Grillo-Lopez AJ, Hedrick E, Rashford M, et al. Rituximab: ongoing and future clinical development. Semin Oncol 2002;29:105–12.

110. Saxena A, Wu D. Advances in therapeutic Fc engineering - modulation of IgG-associated effector functions and serum half-life. Front Immunol 2016;7:580.

111. Weiskopf K, Anderson KL, Ito D, et al. Eradication of canine diffuse large B-cell lymphoma in a murine xenograft model with CD47 blockade and anti-CD20. Cancer Immunol Res 2016;4:1072–87.

112. Jain S, Aresu L, Comazzi S, et al. The development of a recombinant scFv monoclonal antibody targeting canine CD20 for use in comparative medicine. PLoS One 2016;11:e0148366.

113. Ito D, Brewer S, Modiano JF, et al. Development of a novel anti-canine CD20 monoclonal antibody with diagnostic and therapeutic potential. Leuk Lymphoma 2015;56:219–25.

114. Rue SM, Eckelman BP, Efe JA, et al. Identification of a candidate therapeutic antibody for treatment of canine B-cell lymphoma. Vet Immunol Immunopathol 2015;164:148–59.

115. Kano R, Inoiue C, Okano H, et al. Canine CD20 gene. Vet Immunol Immunopathol 2005;108:265–8.

116. Jubala CM, Wojcieszyn JW, Valli VE, et al. CD20 expression in normal canine B cells and in canine non-Hodgkin lymphoma. Vet Pathol 2005;42:468–76.

117. Impellizeri JA, Howell K, McKeever KP, et al. The role of rituximab in the treatment of canine lymphoma: an ex vivo evaluation. Vet J 2006;171:556–8.

118. London CA, Gardner HL, Rippy S, et al. KTN0158, a humanized anti-KIT monoclonal antibody, demonstrates biologic activity against both normal and malignant canine mast cells. Clin Cancer Res 2017;23:2565–74.

119. Adelfinger M, Bessler S, Frentzen A, et al. Preclinical testing oncolytic vaccinia virus strain GLV-5b451 expressing an anti-VEGF single-chain antibody for canine cancer therapy. Viruses 2015;7:4075–92.

120. Wagner S, Maibaum D, Pich A, et al. Verification of a canine PSMA (FolH1) antibody. Anticancer Res 2015;35:145–8.

121. Singer J, Fazekas J, Wang W, et al. Generation of a canine anti-EGFR (ErbB-1) antibody for passive immunotherapy in dog cancer patients. Mol Cancer Ther 2014;13:1777–90.
122. Michishita M, Uto T, Nakazawa R, et al. Antitumor effect of bevacizumab in a xenograft model of canine hemangiopericytoma. J Pharmacol Sci 2013;121: 339–42.
123. Michishita M, Ohtsuka A, Nakahira R, et al. Anti-tumor effect of bevacizumab on a xenograft model of feline mammary carcinoma. J Vet Med Sci 2016;78:685–9.
124. Shahabi V, Seavey MM, Maciag PC, et al. Development of a live and highly attenuated Listeria monocytogenes-based vaccine for the treatment of Her2/neu-overexpressing cancers in human. Cancer Gene Ther 2011;18:53–62.
125. Mason NJ, Gnanandarajah JS, Engiles JB, et al. Immunotherapy with a HER2-targeting listeria induces HER2-specific immunity and demonstrates potential therapeutic effects in a phase I trial in canine osteosarcoma. Clin Cancer Res 2016;22:4380–90.
126. Bergman PJ, Camps-Palau MA, McKnight JA, et al. Development of a xenogeneic DNA vaccine program for canine malignant melanoma at the Animal Medical Center. Vaccine 2006;24(21):4582–5.
127. Bergman PJ, McKnight J, Novosad A, et al. Long-term survival of dogs with advanced malignant melanoma after DNA vaccination with xenogeneic human tyrosinase: a phase I trial. Clin Cancer Res 2003;9(4):1284–90.
128. Smedley RC, Lamoureux J, Sledge DG, et al. Immunohistochemical diagnosis of canine oral amelanotic melanocytic neoplasms. Vet Pathol 2011;48(1):32–40.
129. Phillips JC, Lembcke LM, Noltenius CE, et al. Evaluation of tyrosinase expression in canine and equine melanocytic tumors. Am J Vet Res 2012;73(2):272–8.
130. Cangul IT, van Garderen E, van der Poel HJ, et al. Tyrosinase gene expression in clear cell sarcoma indicates a melanocytic origin: insight from the first reported canine case. APMIS 1999;107(11):982–8.
131. Ramos-Vara JA, Beissenherz ME, Miller MA, et al. Retrospective study of 338 canine oral melanomas with clinical, histologic, and immunohistochemical review of 129 cases. Vet Pathol 2000;37(6):597–608.
132. Ramos-Vara JA, Miller MA. Immunohistochemical identification of canine melanocytic neoplasms with antibodies to melanocytic antigen PNL2 and tyrosinase: comparison with Melan A. Vet Pathol 2011;48(2):443–50.
133. de Vries TJ, Smeets M, de GR, et al. Expression of gp100, MART-1, tyrosinase, and S100 in paraffin-embedded primary melanomas and locoregional, lymph node, and visceral metastases: implications for diagnosis and immunotherapy. A study conducted by the EORTC Melanoma Cooperative Group. J Pathol 2001; 193(1):13–20.
134. Gradilone A, Gazzaniga P, Ribuffo D, et al. Prognostic significance of tyrosinase expression in sentinel lymph node biopsy for ultra-thin, thin, and thick melanomas. Eur Rev Med Pharmacol Sci 2012;16(10):1367–76.
135. Liao JC, Gregor P, Wolchok JD, et al. Vaccination with human tyrosinase DNA induces antibody responses in dogs with advanced melanoma. Cancer Immun 2006;6:8.
136. Goubier A, Fuhrmann L, Forest L, et al. Superiority of needle-free transdermal plasmid delivery for the induction of antigen-specific IFNgamma T cell responses in the dog. Vaccine 2008;26:2186–90.
137. Grosenbaugh DA, Leard AT, Bergman PJ, et al. Safety and efficacy of a xenogeneic DNA vaccine encoding for human tyrosinase as adjunctive treatment

for oral malignant melanoma in dogs following surgical excision of the primary tumor. Am J Vet Res 2011;72(12):1631–8.

138. Herzog A, Buchholz J, Ruess-Melzer K, et al. Combined use of irradiation and DNA tumor vaccine to treat canine oral malignant melanoma: a pilot study. Schweiz Arch Tierheilkd 2013;155(2):135–42 [in German].

139. Ottnod JM, Smedley RC, Walshaw R, et al. A retrospective analysis of the efficacy of Oncept vaccine for the adjunct treatment of canine oral malignant melanoma. Vet Comp Oncol 2013;11(3):219–29.

140. Verganti S, Berlato D, Blackwood L, et al. Use of oncept melanoma vaccine in 69 canine oral malignant melanomas in the UK. J Small Anim Pract 2017;58:10–6.

141. Treggiari E, Grant JP, North SM. A retrospective review of outcome and survival following surgery and adjuvant xenogeneic DNA vaccination in 32 dogs with oral malignant melanoma. J Vet Med Sci 2016;78:845–50.

142. McLean JL, Lobetti RG. Use of the melanoma vaccine in 38 dogs: the South African experience. J S Afr Vet Assoc 2015;86:1246.

143. Boston SE, Lu X, Culp WT, et al. Efficacy of systemic adjuvant therapies administered to dogs after excision of oral malignant melanomas: 151 cases (2001-2012). J Am Vet Med Assoc 2014;245:401–7.

144. Wolchok JD, Yuan J, Houghton AN, et al. Safety and immunogenicity of tyrosinase DNA vaccines in patients with melanoma. Mol Ther 2007;15:2044–50.

145. Perales MA, Yuan J, Powel S, et al. Phase I/II study of GM-CSF DNA as an adjuvant for a multipeptide cancer vaccine in patients with advanced melanoma. Mol Ther 2008;16:2022–9.

146. Yuan J, Ku GY, Gallardo HF, et al. Safety and immunogenicity of a human and mouse gp100 DNA vaccine in a phase I trial of patients with melanoma. Cancer Immun 2009;9:5.

147. Manley CA, Leibman NF, Wolchok JD, et al. Xenogeneic murine tyrosinase DNA vaccine for malignant melanoma of the digit of dogs. J Vet Intern Med 2011; 25(1):94–9.

148. Phillips JC, Blackford JT, Lembcke LM, et al. Evaluation of needle-free injection devices for intramuscular vaccination in horses. J Equine Vet Sci 2011;31: 738–43. Ref Type: Generic.

149. Sarbu L, Kitchell BE, Bergman PJ. Safety of administering the canine melanoma DNA vaccine (Oncept) to cats with malignant melanoma - a retrospective study. J Feline Med Surg 2017;19(2):224–30.

150. Chu PY, Pan SL, Liu CH, et al. KIT gene exon 11 mutations in canine malignant melanoma. Vet J 2013;196(2):226–30.

151. Murakami A, Mori T, Sakai H, et al. Analysis of KIT expression and KIT exon 11 mutations in canine oral malignant melanomas. Vet Comp Oncol 2011;9(3): 219–24.

152. Gillard M, Cadieu E, De BC, et al. Naturally occurring melanomas in dogs as models for non-UV pathways of human melanomas. Pigment Cell Melanoma Res 2014;27(1):90–102.

153. Peggs KS, Quezada SA, Korman AJ, et al. Principles and use of anti-CTLA4 antibody in human cancer immunotherapy. Curr Opin Immunol 2006;18(2): 206–13.

154. Graves SS, Stone D, Loretz C, et al. Establishment of long-term tolerance to SRBC in dogs by recombinant canine CTLA4-Ig. Transplantation 2009;88: 317–22.

155. Callahan MK, Wolchok JD. At the bedside: CTLA-4- and PD-1-blocking antibodies in cancer immunotherapy. J Leukoc Biol 2013;94:41–53.

156. Biller BJ, Elmslie RE, Burnett RC, et al. Use of FoxP3 expression to identify regulatory T cells in healthy dogs and dogs with cancer. Vet Immunol Immunopathol 2007;116:69–78.

157. Horiuchi Y, Tominaga M, Ichikawa M, et al. Increase of regulatory T cells in the peripheral blood of dogs with metastatic tumors. Microbiol Immunol 2009;53: 468–74.

158. O'Neill K, Guth A, Biller B, et al. Changes in regulatory T cells in dogs with cancer and associations with tumor type. J Vet Intern Med 2009;23:875–81.

159. Sherger M, Kisseberth W, London C, et al. Identification of myeloid derived suppressor cells in the peripheral blood of tumor bearing dogs. BMC Vet Res 2012; 8:209.

160. Thamm DH. Interactions between radiation therapy and immunotherapy: the best of two worlds? Vet Comp Oncol 2006;4:189–97.

161. Walter CU, Biller BJ, Lana SE, et al. Effects of chemotherapy on immune responses in dogs with cancer. J Vet Intern Med 2006;20(2):342–7.

162. Emens LA, Jaffee EM. Leveraging the activity of tumor vaccines with cytotoxic chemotherapy. Cancer Res 2005;65(18):8059–64.

163. Wolchok JD, Kluger H, Callahan MK, et al. Nivolumab plus ipilimumab in advanced melanoma. N Engl J Med 2013;369(2):122–33.

164. Ott PA, Hodi FS, Kaufman HL, et al. Combination immunotherapy: a road map. J Immunother Cancer 2017;5:16.

165. Hellmann MD, Friedman CF, Wolchok JD. Combinatorial cancer immunotherapies. Adv Immunol 2016;130:251–77.

166. Le D, Uram J, Wang H, et al. PD-1 blockade in tumors with mismatch-repair deficiency. N Engl J Med 2015;372:2509–20.

167. Karaki S, Anson M, Tran T, et al. Is there still room for cancer vaccines at the era of checkpoint inhibitors. Vaccines (Basel) 2016;4 [pii:E37].

168. Lai X, Friedman A. Combination therapy of cancer with cancer vaccine and immune checkpoint inhibitors: a mathematical model. PLoS One 2017;12: e0178479.

169. Yuasa T, Masuda H, Yamamoto S, et al. Biomarkers to predict prognosis and response to checkpoint inhibitors. Int J Clin Oncol 2017;22:629–34.

170. Khagi Y, Kurzrock R, Patel SP. Next generation predictive biomarkers for immune checkpoint inhibition. Cancer Metastasis Rev 2017;36:179–90.

171. Ott PA, Hu Z, Keskin DB, et al. An immunogenic personal neoantigen vaccine for patients with melanoma. Nature 2017;547:217–21.

172. Jackson HJ, Rafiq S, Brentjens RJ. Driving CAR T-cells forward. Nat Rev Clin Oncol 2016;13:370–83.

173. Coy J, Caldwell A, Chow L, et al. PD-1 expression by canine T cells and functional effects of PD-1 blockade. Vet Comp Oncol 2017;15(4):1487–502.

174. Maekawa N, Konnai S, Okagawa T, et al. Immunohistochemical analysis of PD-L1 expression in canine malignant cancers and PD-1 expression on lymphocytes in canine oral melanoma. PLoS One 2016;11:e0157176.

175. Maekawa N, Konnai S, Takagi S, et al. A canine chimeric monoclonal antibody targeting PD-L1 and its clinical efficacy in canine oral malignant melanoma or undifferentiated sarcoma. Sci Rep 2017;7:8951.

176. Shosu K, Sakurai M, Inoue K, et al. Programmed cell death ligand 1 expression in canine cancer. In Vivo 2016;30:195–204.

177. Chiku VM, Silva KL, de Almeida BF, et al. PD-1 function in apoptosis of T lymphocytes in canine visceral leishmaniasis. Immunobiology 2016;221:879–88.

178. Tagawa M, Maekawa N, Konnai S, et al. Evaluation of costimulatory molecules in peripheral blood lymphocytes of canine patients with histiocytic sarcoma. PLoS One 2016;11:e0150030.

179. Esch KJ, Juelsgaard R, Martinez PA, et al. Programmed death 1-mediated T cell exhaustion during visceral leishmaniasis impairs phagocyte function. J Immunol 2013;191:5542–50.

180. Folkl A, Wen X, Kuczynski E, et al. Feline programmed death and its ligand: characterization and changes with feline immunodeficiency virus infection. Vet Immunol Immunopathol 2010;134:107–14.

181. Kumar SR, Kim DY, Henry CJ, et al. Programmed death ligand 1 is expressed in canine B cell lymphoma and downregulated by MEK inhibitors. Vet Comp Oncol 2017;15(4):1527–36.

182. Smith JB, Panjwani MK, Schutsky K, et al. Feasibility and safety of cCD20 RNA CAR-bearing T cell therapy for the treatment of canine B cell malignancies. J Immunother Cancer 2015;3:123.

183. Anderson KL, Modiano JF. Progress in adaptive immunotherapy for cancer in companion animals: success on the path to a cure. Vet Sci 2015;2:363–87.

184. Mata M, Vera J, Gerken C, et al. Towards immunotherapy with redirected T cells in a large animal model: ex vivo activation, expansion, and genetic modification of canine T cells. J Immunother 2014;37:407–15.

185. Mie K, Shimada T, Akiyoshi H, et al. Change in peripheral blood lymphocyte count in dogs following adoptive immunotherapy using lymphokine-activated T killer cells combined with palliative tumor resection. Vet Immunol Immunopathol 2016;177:58–63.

186. Panjwani MK, Smith JB, Schutsky K, et al. Feasibility and safety of RNA-transfected CD20-specific chimeric antigen receptor T cells in dogs with spontaneous B cell lymphoma. Mol Ther 2016;24:1602–14.

187. Heinzerling L, Goldinger SM. A review of serious adverse effects under treatment with checkpoint inhibitors. Curr Opin Oncol 2017;29:136–44.

188. Kumar V, Chaudhary N, Garg M, et al. Current diagnosis and management of immune related adverse events (irAEs) induced by immune checkpoint inhibitor therapy. Front Pharmacol 2017;8:49.

189. Khanna C, London C, Vail D, et al. Guiding the optimal translation of new cancer treatments from canine to human cancer patients. Clin Cancer Res 2009;15:5671–7.

190. Paoloni M, Khanna C. Translation of new cancer treatments from pet dogs to humans. Nat Rev Cancer 2008;8:147–56.

191. Ranieri G, Gadaleta CD, Patruno R, et al. A model of study for human cancer: spontaneous occurring tumors in dogs. Biological features and translation for new anticancer therapies. Crit Rev Oncol Hematol 2013;88(1):187–97.

192. Angstadt AY, Thayanithy V, Subramanian S, et al. A genome-wide approach to comparative oncology: high-resolution oligonucleotide aCGH of canine and human osteosarcoma pinpoints shared microaberrations. Cancer Genet 2012;205(11):572–87.

193. LeBlanc AK, Breen M, Choyke P, et al. Perspectives from man's best friend: National Academy of Medicine's Workshop on comparative oncology. Sci Transl Med 2016;8:324ps5.

194. LeBlanc AK, Mazcko C, Brown DE, et al. Creation of an NCI comparative brain tumor consortium: informing the translation of new knowledge from canine to human brain tumor patients. Neuro Oncol 2016;18:1209–18.

195. Seelig DM, Avery AC, Ehrhart EJ, et al. The comparative diagnostic features of canine and human lymphoma. Vet Sci 2016;3 [pii:11].
196. Fulkerson CM, Dhawan D, Ratliff TL, et al. Naturally occurring canine invasive urinary bladder cancer: a complementary animal model to improve the success rate in human clinical trials of new cancer drugs. Int J Genomics 2017;2017: 6589529.

Adverse Reactions to Vaccination
From Anaphylaxis to Autoimmunity

 CrossMark

Laurel J. Gershwin, DVM, PhD

KEYWORDS

• Vaccine reactions • IgE • Anaphylaxis • Autoimmunity • Arthus reaction

KEY POINTS

- Vaccines are important for protection of individual animals and for creation of herd immunity against infectious diseases.
- Induction of immune responses to nontarget antigens present in most vaccines can lead to allergic sensitization, particularly in breeds with genetic predisposition.
- Reactions to vaccines can vary from allergic events (face swelling) to anaphylactic shock. Although uncommon, such responses can occur.
- Autoimmune diseases have a variety of causes and generally have a genetic predisposition. Overvaccination in a patient with a predisposition to autoimmune disease may enhance the likelihood for development of an autoimmune response.

Prevention of infectious disease by the use of vaccination is one of the most important procedures performed by veterinarians and human health professionals. In some instances, disease has been completely eradicated or greatly reduced through elicitation of herd immunity. Yet, vaccination is not without risk. A risk of vaccination is associated with misuse, overvaccination, and in a small proportion of the vaccinated population the potential for a potentially fatal allergic reaction exists.

HYPERSENSITIVITY TO VACCINE COMPONENTS

In large and small animal patients administration of a viral vaccine, particularly an inactivated and adjuvanted viral vaccine, can elicit an IgE response to proteins present in the vaccine that are nontarget antigens. These are proteins that are present in the cell culture medium used to grow the virus to be used in the vaccine preparation. If the virus is grown on mammalian cells, the most common nontarget antigens are bovine serum proteins, because of the use of fetal bovine serum in cell growth

The author has nothing to disclose.
Department of Pathology, Microbiology & Immunology, School of Veterinary Medicine, University of California, Davis, Vet Med 3A, One Shields Avenue, Davis, CA 95616, USA
E-mail address: ljgershwin@ucdavis.edu

Vet Clin Small Anim 48 (2018) 279–290
https://doi.org/10.1016/j.cvsm.2017.10.005
0195-5616/18/© 2017 Elsevier Inc. All rights reserved.

vetsmall.theclinics.com

medium. Proteins shed from the cells used to grow the virus are another source of antigen. The actual virus that is the target immunogen is rarely the source of the misdirected immune response. When virus is grown in eggs, some of the egg protein can become a nontarget antigen. In addition, stabilizers, such as gelatin, can occasionally become a target of an unwanted immune response. The process of vaccine production varies with the manufacturer and the type of adjuvant used, but in general it is impossible for the viral antigens to be completely purified so that the tissue culture products are completely eliminated from the final product. For most patients, this is not a problem. Even if a small amount of IgG is made against fetal bovine serum proteins, it is usually harmless. However, in the population of patients with atopy (those that readily make IgE responses and are often allergic) elicitation of an IgE response by these nontarget antigens presents a potential problem.

The presence of the nontarget antigens in multiple viral vaccines means that each time a patient receives a vaccine containing the nontarget antigens those same nontarget antigens are available to restimulate the immune response.

Patients with atopy (dogs, horses) respond to nontarget antigens by making not only IgG but also IgE antibodies. These IgE antibodies have a high affinity for receptors on mast cells in the skin and nearby mucous membranes of the intestinal tract and the respiratory tract. IgE stays on these mast cells for months, even after serum IgE levels have waned. When the patient receives an injection of vaccine containing more nontarget antigens they bind to the IgE on mast cells and cause degranulation. This is a typical type I hypersensitivity response, with liberation of preformed mediators, such as histamine, and stimulation of production of arachidonic acid metabolites by the lipoxygenase and cyclooxygenase pathways. The leukotrienes thereby created along with the released histamine cause vasoactive responses, increased capillary permeability, and even smooth muscle contraction (**Fig. 1**). In the horse and the dog these responses have been shown to be associated with adverse clinical responses. In the horse, one may see signs of colic and in severe instances, respiratory distress and circulatory collapse (anaphylactic shock). In the dog, a common early sign is swelling and urticaria of the muzzle area, with systemic anaphylaxis occurring usually after one or more such episodes of vaccine responses.

These reactions can be startling to owners and veterinarians and can create a dilemma, particularly when giving the required rabies vaccine.

In 1983, Frick and Brooks[1] hypothesized that immunization of dogs with atopy for canine distemper and parvoviruse would alter immunoregulation of the IgE response. An inbred atopic dog colony was used to test this hypothesis. Vaccination of puppies before sensitization with grass and weed pollen extracts seemed to enhance production of IgE antibodies to the pollen allergens.[1]

HogenEsch and colleagues[2] studied a group of Beagles to evaluate the effect of vaccination on serum concentrations of total and antigen-specific IgE. A multivalent vaccine (without adjuvant) failed to alter IgE levels but addition of the rabies vaccine or rabies vaccine alone (containing alum adjuvant) caused there to be an increase in IgE reactive with vaccine antigens. The reactivity of the IgE included the nontarget proteins in the tissue culture fluid: bovine serum albumin and fibronectin.

The possibility that immunization with vaccines containing alum adjuvants would increase IgE antibody levels reactive with allergens to which the patient had already been sensitized was examined by Tater and colleagues.[3] Using a colony of Maltese-Beagle crossbred dogs known to be allergic to corn and soy, the investigators monitored IgE levels specific to these allergens before and after immunization with commonly used vaccines (canine distemper/adenovirus/measles, parvovirus, parainfluenza virus and rabies). In a second experiment the effect of aluminum

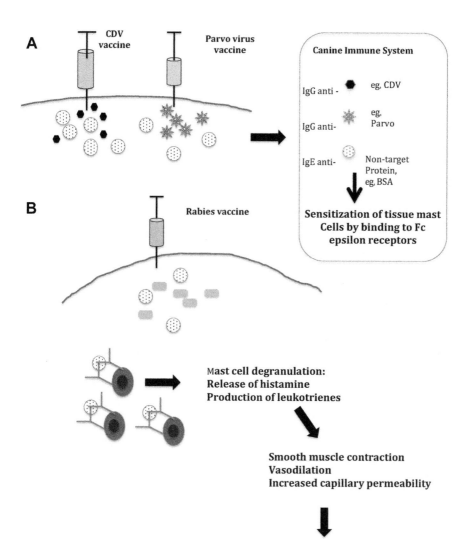

Fig. 1. Viral vaccines contain proteins that are residual from tissue culture media that cop-urify with virus. These are nontarget antigens. (*A*) Administration of a canine distemper vac-cine containing nontarget antigens stimulates the production of antibodies (IgG and sometimes IgE) against the nontarget antigens and against the target viral antigens. The im-mune response to the nontarget antigens is restimulated by any other vaccine containing these antigens, such as Parvovirus vaccine. (*B*) After initiation of an IgE response to nontarget antigens these antibodies bind tightly to tissue mast cells by their Fc receptors. When another vaccine containing nontarget antigens is given, the IgE molecules bind the antigens, cross-linking the Fc receptors, and trigger degranulation of the mast cells. The release of vasoactive mediators, such as histamine, and the initiation of production of the arachidonic acid mediators, prostaglandins and leukotrienes, causes physiologic effects that result in signs of type I hypersensitivity, which may vary from local facial swelling to anaphylactic shock. BSA, bovine serum albumin; CDV, canine distemper vaccine.

hydroxide adjuvant alone on these same parameters was examined. The study concluded that although increases in total IgE were not observed, the vaccination of dogs with these standard vaccines did cause a significant increase in the levels of IgE specific for the corn and soy allergens to which the dogs had been previously sensitized. Inoculation with alum adjuvant alone did not stimulate the specific IgE response.[3] From this study, one can conclude that vaccination of dogs with concurrent allergy may result in worsening of the allergic condition.

A later study by Ohmori and colleagues[4] examined serum from dogs that had reacted adversely to vaccines with clinical signs relevant to anaphylaxis (collapse, facial edema, dyspnea, and vomiting within 1 hour after vaccination). They compared these sera with sera from dogs that did not develop vaccine reactions. The results showed significantly higher IgE levels in dogs that had reacted adversely. Moreover, the IgE reactivity was directed to proteins in fetal bovine serum and to gelatin and casein used as stabilizers.

Our group followed 77 horses for a period of 5 years to determine if yearly vaccination for West Nile virus would induce IgE responses. High, moderate, and non-IgE responders were identified. The reactivity of the IgE was directed predominantly toward nontarget antigens present in the vaccine, horses with the highest levels of IgE reacted to bovine serum albumin, on antigen-specific enzyme-linked immunosorbent assay and by intradermal skin testing.[5] In a subsequent study, we showed that administration of oligodeoxynucleotides containing CpG motifs concurrently with West Nile virus vaccine in high-responder horses increased the numbers of T regulatory cells and concurrently decreased the IgE response; thus, demonstrating a potential strategy for safer immunization of the high-IgE-responder horse.[6]

Adverse reactions to nontarget antigens have also been observed in human patients. In one study of human children in Sri Lanka high levels of IgE specific to bovine serum albumin were detected in those with measles vaccine allergy.[7] Other reports describe mumps-measles-rubella and/or influenza vaccine reactions in patients with egg allergy caused by growth of the target virus in eggs and the incorporation of ovalbumin in the vaccine as a nontarget antigen.[8] Overall the incidence of vaccine reactions in human patients with egg allergy is low.

TESTING FOR POTENTIAL VACCINE REACTIVITY

The requirement for rabies vaccination is problematic for owners of dogs that have shown allergic reactivity to vaccines. Requirements vary by state and the substitution of a serum antibody titer against rabies virus may be acceptable. One possible method to determine if a vaccine is likely to elicit an adverse (IgE mediated) response is to perform an intradermal skin test using the vaccine. This simple test may allow the veterinarian to select a product that is less likely to elicit allergic reactivity in a sensitive patient. To perform the test, 0.1 mL of the vaccine is injected by the intradermal route into shaven skin on the lateral thorax. Similar injections are performed with the diluent (or sterile saline solution) as a negative control and histamine as a positive control. Injection sites are observed and wheal development is measured after 15 to 20 minutes. The presence of a wheal at the vaccine site indicates a positive response to the vaccine, that is, the vaccine contains one or more antigens that are able to stimulate IgE present on tissue mast cells of the patient.

LOCAL VACCINE REACTIONS: ARTHUS REACTION

Although the immediate type I IgE-mediated responses to vaccine-associated nontarget allergens can be serious, a less serious, but annoying response to vaccination can also occur. The Arthus reaction is mediated by immune complexes, a typical type III hypersensitivity response.[9] Typically the Arthus reaction occurs within 24 hours after the vaccine is given and is localized to the injection site. The area becomes swollen and painful. On histologic examination the tissue shows vasculitis with infiltration of neutrophils. Sometimes local hemorrhage can also be a feature of this response. These responses occur because there is circulating IgG, specific for either target or nontarget antigens. When more antigen is injected into the tissue, immune complexes form within and around dermal blood vessels. Fixation of complement by these complexes causes production of chemotactic factors, C3a and C5a, which cause degranulation of mast cells and neutrophil chemotaxis (**Fig. 2**). The resulting inflammation leads to swelling and pain in the area. Generally after 2 to 3 days the lesion resolves. However, the lesson learned is often that the patient is not likely to need another booster immunization in the near future (if an older patient, possibly not at all). Determination of a titer against the vaccine target antigen is a logical step toward deciding when and if to revaccinate the patient. The Arthus reaction should be differentiated from an adjuvant reaction.

FELINE VACCINE–ASSOCIATED FIBROSARCOMA

Like vaccine-induced anaphylaxis the development of fibrosarcomas in response to vaccination in cats is rare (estimated between 1 in 1000 and 1 in 10,000 vaccinated cats).[10] Nonetheless, if the cat affected is your patient or your pet, that statistic is not particularly comforting. The development of fibrosarcoma at the injection site of a vaccine began being recognized in 1991. Administration of adjuvanted killed vaccines (rabies and feline leukemia) is associated with development of these tumors.[10] Over the years a variety of studies have been performed to determine the cause of the response, and associated host and vaccine factors. In 1996 a Vaccine Associated Feline Sarcoma Task Force was initiated with resultant changes in feline vaccine protocols and procedures. A nonadjuvanted rabies vaccine for cats subsequently became available but according to a recent study in Canada, the incidence of post-vaccine fibrosarcomas has not shown a significant decline.[10]

One result of the recognition of vaccine-associated fibrosarcomas in cats has been an effort to put vaccines in specific sites, such as feline leukemia as far down on the left leg as possible, and rabies as far down on the right leg as possible. This process serves two purposes: to determine which vaccine is causal in the event that a tumor does occur, and to make it possible to save an animal's life by leg amputation should a tumor occur. Administration of vaccines in the intrascapular area makes it nearly impossible to surgically remove tumors in that site.

VACCINE-INDUCED DISEASE EXACERBATION: A BARRIER TO VACCINE DEVELOPMENT

When patients who have been vaccinated against a particular pathogen are exposed to that pathogen, if the vaccine is effective the patient should either not develop the disease or perhaps develop only a mild form of the disease. There are some instances in which a vaccine not only failed to protect but actually caused a more severe disease than would be expected in an unvaccinated patient. The cause of vaccine-induced disease enhancement is induction of an immune response that is pathogenic rather than protective. This type of response has been documented first in human children inoculated with formalin-inactivated alum adjuvanted respiratory syncytial virus vaccine, then in bovine respiratory syncytial virus vaccinated calves.[11] Research has shown that in the latter case the killed vaccine stimulates a strong T-helper type 2 response, with predominant interleukin (IL)-4 production and IgE antibodies directed

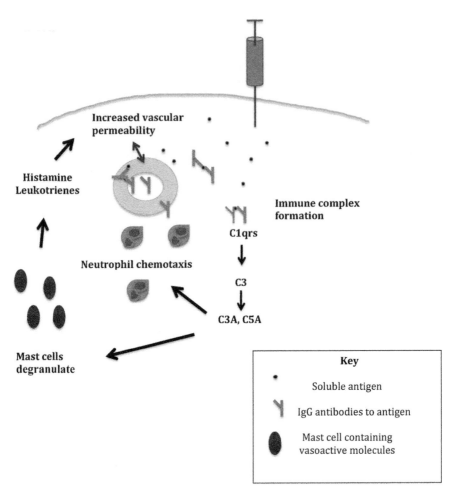

Fig. 2. The clinical syndrome called the Arthus reaction results from a localized type III hypersensitivity reaction. The Arthus reaction is usually seen in animals that have been vaccinated many times (eg, an older dog that has had yearly vaccines for many years). In the patient that has made high levels of IgG antibodies to the vaccine antigens, there is IgG in the interstitial tissue fluids and in the blood. When the vaccine antigens are introduced they bind to the antibodies creating immune complexes, complement is fixed, and C3a and C5a are produced. These small by-products of complement fixation cause mast cells to degranulate and release histamine with consequent increased permeability of the local blood vessels, allowing more IgG to leave the blood vessels and allowing immune complexes to penetrate the vessel walls. Chemotaxis of neutrophils is also stimulated by these chemotactic factors and an accumulation of neutrophils occurs in the area of the injection. The end result is an inflamed, swollen area that appears hours after the injection and can last for several days.

against viral proteins.[12] For viral clearance the more effective immune response is a T-helper type 1 response, with production of interferon gamma. Research performed using cotton rats and mice as models have shown that when the immune system's first encounter with the respiratory syncytial virus/bovine respiratory syncytial virus is with the killed virion, modulation of the immune response favors the T-helper type 2 response; whereas when that first encounter is with live (or a living attenuated) virus a more balanced immune response results. Recent research on respiratory syncytial virus vaccination using a cotton rat model has shown that when the viral antigen is inert (eg, a subunit fusion protein) the dose is an important factor that determines whether vaccine exacerbation occurs.[13] Our group found that to also be true for the formalin inactivated alum adjuvanted bovine respiratory syncytial virus vaccine.[12]

Feline infectious peritonitis (FIP) is another disease that has been associated with vaccine-induced enhancement. FIP is caused by a coronavirus, which is thought to have mutated from the common feline enteric coronavirus. The pathogenesis of FIP is complex, but the most recent data suggest that macrophages play an important role in harboring and propagating the virus.[14] A vaccine for FIP that was previously on the market induced IgG against the virus, which for many infectious agents would be protective. However, for FIP these antibodies opsonized virions for enhanced phagocytosis by macrophages, thus facilitating spread of the virus within the cat. As with dengue, a tropical disease affecting humans, FIP is also associated with antibody-dependent enhancement of disease. In the presence of nonneutralizing IgG human patients infected with dengue virus can progress to hemorrhagic fever or dengue shock syndrome.[15] The currently accepted explanation for this pathogenesis involves opsonization of the virus by the nonneutralizing IgG with subsequent immune complex binding to Fc receptors and enhanced cell infection caused by improved phagocytosis. Cats infected with FIP virus type I and passively immunized with FIP antibody against virus type 2 had a significantly lower survival rate than cats that did not receive the passive antibody.[16] The spike protein (S) is the target for neutralizing antibody production. A recombinant vaccinia virus vectored vaccine containing the gene coding for the S protein was tested in kittens subsequently infected with virulent FIP. Vaccinated kittens died earlier than similarly infected control kittens.[17] In another study DNA vaccination was used to attempt to induce a cell-mediated immune response to FIP virus. Codelivery of plasmids containing IL-12 and the nucleocapsid (N) and membrane protein (M) was used in a prime-boost schedule before virulent FIP challenge. The infected kittens that received the vaccine containing the IL-12 gene had a shorter survival time that those receiving the plasmid coding for the two FIP antigens (N and M) without the IL-12, thus suggesting some degree of enhancement.[18]

VACCINATION AND AUTOIMMUNITY

In recent years there has been much conjecture and some case histories that suggest a possible connection between overstimulation of the immune response with excessive vaccination and the development of autoimmune disease, such as immune-mediated anemia. Evidence for this is scant but there are a few studies that substantiate a connection. A controlled retrospective study on dogs that developed immune-mediated hemolytic anemia (IMHA) compared dogs that developed IMHA within a month after vaccination with dogs that developed IMHA more than a month after vaccination. The study found that a significant number of the 58 study dogs (26%) had developed IMHA within a month of vaccination. The mean number of days postvaccination was 13 days. In contrast the control group of dogs did not show an association between vaccination and development of IMHA. The vaccines used in this study were common: distemper, hepatitis, parvovirus, leptospirosis bacterin, and *Bordetella bronchiseptica* bacterin from a variety of pharmaceutical suppliers. The authors conclude that their study defines a temporal association between vaccination of dogs with commonly used vaccines and development of IMHA.[19] In contrast, there are several other published studies that fail to associate vaccination with development of IMHA in dogs. These include a study by Carr and colleagues[20] in which a group of 72 dogs with IMHA were compared with 29 dogs in a vaccine control group. No significant differences were found when the temporal relationship between vaccination and initiation of disease was examined.

Autoimmune diseases in dogs are associated with certain genetic haplotypes[21] and thus it is not surprising that one sees more autoimmune disease in certain breeds. For example, the Samoyed has a much higher[21] chance of developing diabetes mellitus than most other breeds. Autoimmune thyroiditis is more common in the Labrador retrievers. Although there are some autoimmune diseases for which there is a direct connection to a particular infection or other instigating factor, in most cases the factors that contribute to the development of an autoimmune response are likely multiple and for the most part unknown.

The notion that vaccination causes autoimmunity is almost certainly false. However, it is likely that a combination of genetics, environmental factors, and overstimulation of the immune system (which can occur as a result of overvaccination) contribute to development of many autoimmune diseases. It is not uncommon to hear a case history of a middle-aged dog who has had yearly vaccines since puppyhood develop acute hemolytic anemia 2 weeks after a visit to her veterinarian for annual booster vaccination. In such a patient stimulation of a "cytokine storm" by multiple vaccine antigens and adjuvants could provide T-cell help to B cells that are self-reactive, but normally kept in check as a result of the absence of T-cell help. The concept of bystander cell activation has been suggested as a potential result of overstimulation of the immune system by injection of multiple vaccines at once as often as every 6 to 12 months. Cytokine production in the localized microenvironment of lymphoid tissues may lead to promiscuous stimulation of potentially autoreactive B cells. Self-tolerance is achieved by the removal of self-reactive T cells in the thymus during fetal development, but tolerance at the level of the B cell is often maintained because of the absence of T-cell help. Acquisition of T-cell help by self-reactive B cells may cause autoantibody production and subsequent autoimmune disease.[22]

In one study the presence of antithyroglobulin antibodies after routine vaccination was examined in pet dogs and research Beagles. Hypothyroidism is one of the more common autoimmune diseases in humans and dogs; it is estimated that about 50% of hypothyroid dogs have autoimmune thyroiditis. In this study 20 research dogs and 16 pet dogs were followed after vaccination with multivalent vaccine with or without rabies vaccine. The research dogs were vaccinated seven times until 52 weeks of age and then every 6 months until 4 years of age (much more frequently than recommended). The pet dogs were all older than 2 years of age and received a booster vaccine and were checked 14 days later. A thyroid profile consisting of T4 and thyroid-stimulating hormone levels and baseline complete blood count and blood chemistry was performed. In addition, antibodies to bovine and canine thyroglobulin were evaluated. Antibovine and anticanine thyroglobulin antibodies were found in sera from vaccinated dogs. In the pet dogs the anticanine thyroglobulin antibodies were significantly increased and those specific to bovine thyroglobulin were not. The dogs that received the multivalent vaccine without the killed alum adjuvanted rabies vaccine did not show a significant increase in antithyroglobulin antibodies when compared with unvaccinated control animals, but dogs that received the rabies vaccine showed a significant difference from those groups that did not receive the rabies vaccine. There is no known correlate with the development of autoimmune thyroiditis and the role of antibody in pathogenesis of canine Hashimoto's thyroiditis is still being debated. However, the authors suggest that the presence of bovine thyroglobulin in the fetal bovine serum used to assist cell culture propagation may play a role in vaccine-induced stimulation of this immune response.[23] Stimulation of antibodies to canine thyroglobulin by immunization with bovine thyroglobulin (inadvertently as a vaccine nontarget antigen) could solicit T-cell help for self-reactive B cells by exposure to cross-reactive epitopes (**Fig. 3**).

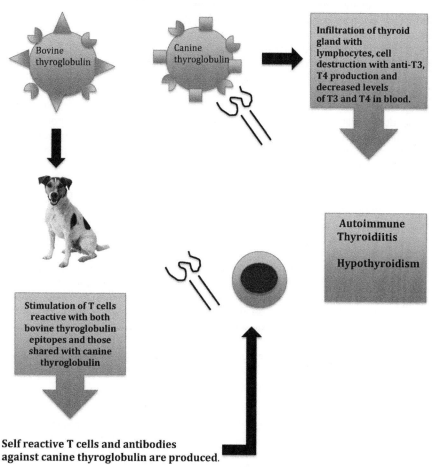

Vaccination with viral vaccine eg, rabies, canine distemper virus, canine parvovirus grown in tissue culture media contaminated with bovine proteins from fetal bovine serum

Bovine thyroglobulin

Canine thyroglobulin

Infiltration of thyroid gland with lymphocytes, cell destruction with anti-T3, T4 production and decreased levels of T3 and T4 in blood.

Autoimmune Thyroidiitis

Hypothyroidism

Stimulation of T cells reactive with both bovine thyroglobulin epitopes and those shared with canine thyroglobulin

Self reactive T cells and antibodies against canine thyroglobulin are produced.

Fig. 3. Autoimmune thyroiditis (Hashimoto's thyroiditis) occurs when activated T lymphocytes attack the thyroid gland and cause cell necrosis. The production of antibodies specific for thyroid antigens is usually another feature of the disease. The resulting destruction of the glandular tissue causes a lack of the thyroid hormones, thyroxin (T3, T4), and with it clinical signs relevant to the hypothyroid state. One hypothesis as to how this occurs is that the presence of bovine thyroglobulin in vaccines (nontarget antigen) stimulates a cross-reactive epitope in the canine thyroid and recruits autoreactive T cells, which then mediate the immune destruction. The disease is more common in certain dog breeds; thus, genetics undoubtedly influences this response.

GENETICS AND AUTOIMMUNITY

The link between autoimmune disease and genetics is well established. For example, it is known that if a person has the major histocompatibility complex B27 allele he or she has a strong likelihood of developing the autoimmune disease ankylosing spondylitis.[22] Canine histocompatibility antigens (DLA) have been linked to a variety of autoimmune diseases. The relative risk of developing many of the currently recognized autoimmune diseases of dogs is higher in dogs with certain DLA haplotypes.[21] The notable increased incidence of particular autoimmune diseases in specific breeds has led to analysis of DLA haplotype associations. The high incidence of diabetes mellitus in Samoyed dogs compared with the rare occurrence of this disease in the Boxer breed led to an evaluation of 460 cases and 1047 controls which revealed a DLA DQ haplotype that was significantly reduced in cases with diabetes mellitus.[24] In another study Cocker Spaniels, a breed with an increased incidence of IMHA, were evaluated for DLA haplotype DLA-DQB1 prevalence of IMHA. Affected and unaffected Cocker Spaniels were evaluated and no significant difference was identified.[25] However, other studies have identified in German Shepherd dogs and Pembroke Welsh Corgis that DLA-DQB1 duplication is a risk allele for exocrine pancreatic insufficiency.[26] Nova Scotia duck tolling retrievers are predisposed to an immune-mediated disease resembling systemic lupus erythematosus in humans. An association with a DLA class II haplotype was found to be highly significant for the development of the lupus-like syndrome in homozygous dogs.[27]

In recent years the veterinary profession has taken a closer look at the duration of immunity for core canine and feline vaccines. Studies have been published that confirm a longer duration of immunity that lasts for at least 3 years for core vaccines. This information has instigated a change in vaccination recommendations: the American Veterinary Medical Association, American Animal Hospital Association, and the Association of Feline Practitioners have all determined that after puppy/kitten vaccines and a 1-year booster, in subsequent years core vaccines need be given only every 3 years. This schedule is expected to reduce the unnecessary immune stimulation and if frequent vaccination is a factor in development of autoimmunity, the incidence of these diseases may be expected to decrease. Increasing research to create better knowledge of the genetic predispositions for autoimmune disease in particular dog breeds coupled with alterations in patterns of vaccination will likely be the key to prevention of an adverse interaction between vaccine practices and canine genetic factors.

SUMMARY

In this article a variety of potential detrimental effects of vaccination are described. It is important for veterinarians to be aware of these for appropriate modification of immunization schemes for individual patients as needed. However, it must be emphasized that the number of pets that suffer from vaccine reactions is extremely low and that most available vaccines are safe and efficacious. Vaccination of animal companions is an important part of an overall health program and should be conducted according to the current standards.

REFERENCES

1. Frick OL, Brooks DL. Immunoglobulin E antibodies to pollens augmented in dogs by virus vaccines. Am J Vet Res 1983;44(3):440–5.

2. HogenEsch H, Dunham AD, Scott-Moncrieff C, et al. Effect of vaccination on serum concentrations of total and antigen specific immunoglobulin E in dogs. Am J Vet Res 2002;63(4):611–6.

3. Tater KC, Jackson HA, Paps J, et al. Effects of routine prophylactic vaccination or administration of aluminum adjuvant alone on allergen-specific serum IgE and IgG responses in allergic dogs. Am J Vet Res 2005;66(9):1572–7.

4. Ohmori K, Masuda K, Maeda S, et al. IgE reactivity to vaccine components in dogs that developed immediate-type allergic reactions after vaccination. Vet Immunol Immunopathol 2005;104(3–4):249–56.

5. Gershwin LJ, Netherwood KA, Norris MS, et al. Equine IgE responses to non-viral vaccine components. Vaccine 2012;30(52):7615–20.

6. Behrens NE, Gershwin LJ. Immune modulation of T regulatory cells and IgE responses in horses vaccinated with West Nile virus vaccine combined with a CpG ODN. Vaccine 2015;33(43):5764–71.

7. de Silva R, Dasanayake WM, Wickramasinhe GD, et al. Sensitization to bovine serum albumin as a possible cause of allergic reactions to vaccines. Vaccine 2017;35(11):1494–500.

8. Chernin LR, Swender D, Hostoffer RW Jr. Cracking the shell on egg-hypersensitive patients and egg-containing vaccines. J Am Osteopath Assoc 2011;111(10 Suppl 6):S5–6.

9. Tizard I. Veterinary Immunology. Chapter 30. 9th edition. Philadelphia: Saunders; 2013.

10. Wilcock B, Wilcock A, Bottoms K. Feline postvaccinal sarcoma: 20 years later. Can Vet J 2012;53(4):430–4.

11. Gershwin LJ, Schelegle ES, Gunther RA, et al. A bovine model of vaccine enhanced respiratory syncytial virus pathophysiology. Vaccine 1998;16(11–12): 1225–36.

12. Kalina WV, Woolums AR, Berghaus RD, et al. Formalin-inactivated bovine RSV vaccine enhances a Th2 mediated immune response in infected cattle. Vaccine 2004;22(11–12):1465–74.

13. Schneider-Ohrum K, Cayatte C, Bennett AS, et al. Immunization with low doses of recombinant postfusion or prefusion respiratory syncytial virus F primes for vaccine-enhanced disease in the cotton rat model independently of the presence of a Th1-biasing (GLA-SE) or Th2-biasing (Alum) adjuvant. J Virol 2017;91(8) [pii: e02180-16].

14. Tekes G, Thiel HJ. Feline coronaviruses: pathogenesis of feline infectious peritonitis. Adv Virus Res 2016;96:193–218.

15. Wang TT, Sewatanon J, Memoli MJ, et al. IgG antibodies to dengue enhanced for FcγRIIIA binding determine disease severity. Science 2017;355(6323):395–8.

16. Takano T, Kawakami C, Yamada S, et al. Antibody-dependent enhancement occurs upon re-infection with the identical serotype virus in feline infectious peritonitis virus infection. J Vet Med Sci 2008;70(12):1315–21.

17. Venneme H, de Groot RJ, Harbour DA, et al. Early death after feline infectious peritonitis virus challenge due to recombinant vaccinia virus immunization. J Virol 1990;64:1407–9.

18. Glansbeek HL, Haagmans BL, te Lintelo EG, et al. Adverse effects of feline IL-12 during DNA vaccination against feline infectious peritonitis virus. J Gen Virol 2002;83(Pt 1):1–10.

19. Duval D, Giger U. Vaccine-associated immune-mediated hemolytic anemia in the dog. J Vet Intern Med 1996;10(5):290–5.

20. Carr AP, Panciera DL, Kidd L. Prognostic factors for mortality and thromboembolism in canine immune-mediated hemolytic anemia: a retrospective study of 72 dogs. J Vet Intern Med 2002;16(5):504–9.
21. Tizard IR. Veterinary immunology. Chapter 34. 9th edition. Philadelphia: Saunders; 2013.
22. Murphy K, Weaver C. Janeway's immunobiology. 9th edition. Garland Sciences; 2016.
23. Scott-Moncrieff JC, Azcona-Olivera J, Glickman NW, et al. Evaluation of antithyroglobulin antibodies after routine vaccination in pet and research dogs. J Am Vet Med Assoc 2002;221(4):515–21.
24. Kennedy LJ, Davison LJ, Barnes A, et al. Identification of susceptibility and protective major histocompatibility complex haplotypes in canine diabetes mellitus. Tissue Antigens 2006;68(6):467–76.
25. Threlfall AJ, Boag AM, Soutter F, et al. Analysis of DLA-DQB1 and polymorphisms in CTLA4 in Cocker spaniels affected with immune-mediated haemolytic anaemia. Canine Genet Epidemiol 2015;2:8.
26. Evans JM, Tsai KL, Starr-Moss AN, et al. Association of DLA-DQB1 alleles with exocrine pancreatic insufficiency in Pembroke Welsh Corgis. Anim Genet 2015; 46(4):462–5.
27. Wilbe M, Jokinen P, Hermanrud C, et al. MHC class II polymorphism is associated with a canine SLE-related disease complex. Immunogenetics 2009;61(8):557–64.

Vaccines in Shelters and Group Settings

Richard A. Squires, BVSc, PhD

KEYWORDS

- Dogs • Cats • Vaccines • Vaccinations • Animal shelters • Rescue shelters
- Shelter medicine

KEY POINTS

- Animals living or congregating in medium-sized to large groups are at much greater risk of acquiring 1 or more contagious infectious diseases than animals living alone or in small groups. They need protecting.
- Special recommendations for the vaccination of young animals in group situations, especially those housed in animal shelters, have been published. These generally recommend an earlier start to vaccination, more frequent vaccination while maternal antibodies are likely to be interfering with immunization, and a slightly later finish.
- Adult animals entering such facilities or engaging in group activities also need the protection of vaccination if their previous vaccination status is uncertain.

INTRODUCTION

Population size, density, and instability have long been recognized as crucially important determinants of the risk of acquiring contagious infectious diseases.[1,2] So, special consideration of the use of vaccines in animal shelters and other group settings is appropriate. Many animal shelters contain large, rapidly fluctuating populations of variably disease-susceptible animals in high-density housing. Many, although certainly not all, must operate with less-than-optimal resourcing. It is extremely challenging to limit contagious infectious diseases in such facilities. Vaccines play an important role in an overarching shelter management strategy that is intended to limit morbidity and mortality in individual animals, and to avoid or minimize the frequency of disease outbreaks while (crucially) enabling the shelter to continue to fulfill its overall mission and goals for society.[3]

This article focuses on the use of vaccines in dogs and cats that are housed or congregate in groups, especially those living in animal shelters. Only vaccines

Disclosure Statement: Dr R.A. Squires is a member of the WSAVA Vaccination Guidelines Group, a group of independent academics whose travel is sponsored by MSD Animal Health.
Veterinary Clinical Sciences, Veterinary Science, Discipline of Veterinary Science, James Cook University, 1 Solander Road, Townsville, Queensland 4811, Australia
E-mail address: Richard.Squires@jcu.edu.au

intended to help prevent or diminish the severity of contagious infectious diseases are considered.

EXISTING GUIDELINES FOR THE USE OF VACCINES IN ANIMAL SHELTERS

Several large veterinary professional organizations have, over the last 2 decades, produced periodically updated guidelines and recommendations for the vaccination of dogs and cats.[4–8] To a large extent, the recommendations provided by these organizations are in agreement with each another.[9] Links to the most recent of these guidelines are provided in **Table 1**. All of these organizations provide separate, specific advice concerning the use of vaccines in animal shelters, either as separate publications[7,10] or embedded in their main guidelines documents.[4]

Quality and Volume of Available Evidence to Guide Decision-Making

Although multiple sets of detailed, increasingly well-referenced guidelines exist, it should be recognized that the quality of available scientific evidence on which vaccination guidelines are based is variable, the total quantity of evidence remains quite limited, and some of the evidence is not readily accessible by veterinary scientists and clinicians. By no means is all of the evidence peer reviewed and, in any case, peer review cannot be relied on as an absolute guarantee of scientific rigor and reliability. As a consequence, at least 1 of the organizations that produce vaccination guidelines has developed a framework that categorizes the quality of evidence provided by publications in veterinary vaccinology.[4] This categorization is useful; inevitably, however, there is substantial variability in quality and reliability within each of the defined categories.

VACCINES NEED TO FIT WITHIN AN OVERALL HEALTH MANAGEMENT PROGRAM IN AN ANIMAL SHELTER

Animal shelters in America have an interesting history, having evolved from livestock impounds that were established in colonial villages and towns.[11] Today's animal shelters are enormously variable in almost every conceivable way (eg, mission, goals, governance, philosophic approach, management, size, design, funding, staffing, community involvement, and location). Despite this enormous heterogeneity, shelters grapple with many shared challenges.[3]

Table 1
Organizations that have published vaccination guidelines over the last 2 decades, including specific recommendations for vaccination of animals in shelters

Name of Organization	Publication Dates for Guidelines	Species Covered	Link to Their Most Recent Guidelines
AAFP	1998, 2000, 2006, 2013	Cats	https://www.catvets.com/guidelines/practice-guidelines/feline-vaccination-guidelines
AAHA	2003, 2006, 2007, 2011, 2017	Dogs	https://www.aaha.org/guidelines/canine_vaccination_guidelines.aspx
WSAVA	2007, 2010, 2016	Both	http://www.wsava.org/guidelines/vaccination-guidelines
ABCD	2009, 2013, 2015	Cats	http://www.abcdcatsvets.org/guidelines/

Abbreviations: AAFP, American Association of Feline Practitioners; AAHA, American Animal Hospital Association; ABCD, European Advisory Board on Cat Diseases; WSAVA, World Small Animal Veterinary Association.

Typically, shelters are facilities that house animals for a variable period of time, usually while the animals are awaiting adoption or reclamation by their owners. There is a high throughput, or population turnover, in many shelters. The animals that arrive are of varying age, sex, health status, geographic origin, prior exposure to infectious agents, and susceptibility to infection. Many have a completely unknown vaccination history (and should be assumed to be unprotected). Some will be fully susceptible to important contagious diseases, whereas others will be currently infected and shedding. Yet others will have been previously infected or vaccinated and will now be robustly immune. Young animals (<4–5 months) may be passively protected against certain diseases by maternal antibodies but will, in the near future, become fully susceptible.

In a recently published report,[12] 41.2% of 51 dogs (≥4 months of age) arriving at a shelter in Indianapolis were seropositive to canine distemper virus (CDV) and 84.3% were seropositive to canine parvovirus (CPV). In a second report describing 431 dogs arriving at a Florida animal shelter, 35.5% of dogs were seropositive to both CDV and CPV, 7.7% to CDV only, 31.5% to CPV only, and 25.3% to neither virus.[13] Older dogs were more likely to have positive antibody titers to both viruses and neutered dogs were more likely to be immune to CDV. It is unknown how many of the dogs in these 2 studies had been naturally exposed or vaccinated. Neutered animals had clearly undergone at least 1 significant veterinary intervention and could be expected to have also been vaccinated. Persistence of passive, maternally derived antibodies is also a possibility in some of the youngest of these dogs.

Cats and kittens entering shelters may also be seropositive to vaccine-preventable infectious disease agents. DiGangi and colleagues[14] studied 347 cats (≥8 weeks) in Florida and reported seropositivity to feline panleukopenia virus (FPV) (39.8%), feline herpesvirus (FHV)-1 (11%), and feline calicivirus (FCV) (36.6%). Thus, in both cats and dogs, a large proportion of animals entering shelters should be considered (based on antibody titers) to be unprotected against vaccine-preventable diseases, supporting current recommendations to vaccinate all animals at (or preferably before) admission into the shelter facility.

This article is focused on the use of vaccines in shelters; however, it is crucial to recognize that each shelter requires a sophisticated, integrated health care program that takes into consideration the points made previously, as well as many others, and ranges far beyond consideration of mere vaccines and parasiticides. **Fig. 1** attempts to itemize some of the factors that interact and influence the effectiveness of vaccines and vaccination programs when these are used in shelters.

VACCINATION OF DOGS AND CATS IN SHELTERS

Guidelines[5,6,8] and textbooks[15,16] recommend that cats, kittens, puppies, and dogs should be vaccinated immediately on entry to the shelter (and preferably before) against the following core infectious agents.

Vaccinations for kittens and cats
- FPV
- FCV
- FHV-1.

Vaccinations for puppies and dogs
- CDV
- Canine adenovirus (CAV)-1 and CAV-2 (using a vaccine containing CAV-2)
- CPV-2 and its variant forms.

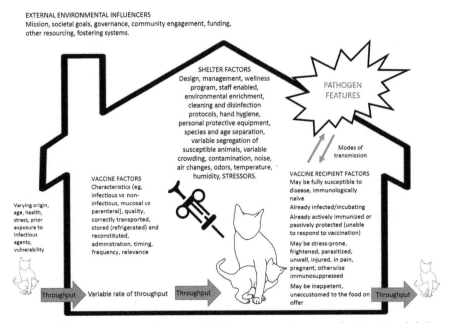

EXTERNAL ENVIRONMENTAL INFLUENCERS
Mission, societal goals, governance, community engagement, funding, other resourcing, fostering systems.

Fig. 1. Vaccines are only part of an overall infection control strategy for the animal shelter. Attention must be paid to factors that directly and indirectly help diminish vaccine recipients' susceptibility to infectious disease and that diminish exposure to pathogens. For example, parasitism may diminish disease resistance and should be addressed, along with vaccination, at the time of admission. Pathogen features that may limit or prevent successful immunization by vaccination are itemized in **Box 1**.

It is also highly recommended, if resources permit, to vaccinate puppies against these respiratory pathogens:

- *Bordetella bronchiseptica* (Bb)
- Canine parainfluenza virus (CPiV).

It is also highly recommended, if cats will be group-housed, to vaccinate them against feline leukemia virus (FeLV).

The onset of a degree of protection can be remarkably swift after vaccination, much earlier than many veterinarians realize.[17] It is widely held that intranasal vaccines

---

Box 1
Pathogen features that limit or prevent successful immunization by vaccination

- Infectious particles are shed in large numbers relative to infectious dose
- Infectious particles are shed by animals that are showing no clinical signs
- Resists most disinfectants
- Does not induce long-lasting protection, even after natural infection
- Nursing mothers typically transfer to kittens or puppies large amounts of antibody against this agent, leading to remarkably long-lasting maternal interference with vaccination
- Infection typically happens very early in life, usually before the animal reaches the shelter

against Bb and CPiV begin to provide mucosal immune protection rapidly, within 72 hours of dosing, although the quality of some of the evidence supporting this contention has recently been contested.[18] It is less well known that subcutaneously injected modified live virus (MLV) vaccines against CPV, FPV, and CDV are also reported to begin to provide protection remarkably early, in situations in which interfering maternal antibodies are not preventing development of an active immune response in the young animal.[17,19]

The question of how early young puppies and kittens can be vaccinated is of practical importance and often raised. Mucosal vaccines (eg, intranasal Bb vaccines) are safe for use in very young puppies and not inactivated by passively transferred maternal antibodies. These can thus be used, with an expectation of success, in young puppies, as early as 3 to 4 weeks of age. Recombinant CDV vaccines do not contain whole, attenuated CDV and may thus be safer for use in very young puppies than are conventional MLV CDV vaccines. These can also be used early, although passively transferred maternal antibodies (less prone to interfere with recombinant vaccines) may nevertheless render them ineffective when used at an early age. The other parenterally administered MLV vaccines or vaccine components are not safe for use before the puppy or kitten reaches 4 weeks of age.

Puppies and kittens from 4 to 20 weeks of age present a special challenge in the shelter because passively transferred maternal antibodies interfere with vaccine efficacy variably. In an individual animal, it is impossible to predict (without testing) which vaccine dose will actually immunize. This is because the amount of antibodies transferred from mother to offspring, mostly in colostrum, varies from individual to individual, and from disease agent to disease agent.[20] Titer testing every puppy or kitten would be expensive and time-consuming. In addition, titer testing of kittens and cats is far less informative than in dogs.[6]

A recommended approach to this dilemma is to vaccinate puppies and kittens repeatedly during this critical period, every 2 to 3 weeks (**Tables 2** and **3** for details). Whether to choose 2 or 3 weeks depends on the intensity of disease challenge and the funds available. It has been recommended[15] to not vaccinate these young animals more often than every 2 weeks, even if that is affordable, because such frequent vaccination is reported to have the opposite of the desired effect, potentially weakening the active immune response and increasing the risk of adverse reactions.

Guidelines[4,6,8] and textbooks[15] differ slightly in their recommendations about when to inject the last vaccine dose to puppies and kittens in the shelter situation. World Small Animal Veterinary Association (WSAVA) recommends that 2 weekly injections continue until 20 weeks of age, whereas American Animal Hospital Association (AAHA) recommends 2 to 3 weekly injections until 18 to 20 weeks. These differences are minor and merely reflect different degrees of risk tolerance, rather than fundamental differences in understanding of underlying immunology. Shelters will be guided by local circumstances and perhaps fluctuating intensity of disease pressure.

Adult dogs or puppies older than about 20 weeks of age can be immunized with a single dose of MLV or recombinant vaccine against CDV, CPV, and CAV-1 and CAV-2. In contrast, it is recommended that cats older than 20 weeks receive 2 doses, 2 to 4 weeks apart, to protect against FHV-1 and FCV. A single dose is sufficient to protect these cats against FPV. If irrefutable evidence of vaccination is provided for an adult animal at the time of admission to a shelter, there is no reason to revaccinate with canine core vaccines, but feline core vaccines, specifically FCV and FHV-1, may be of value in boosting immunity.

Table 2
Recommendations derived by review of American Animal Hospital Association[8] and World Small Animal Veterinary Association[4] guidelines for vaccination of puppies and dogs entering and living in shelters

Vaccine	Puppies ≤18–20 wk	Puppies >18 wk and Adults	Comments
CDV + CAV-2 + CPV ± CPiV (MLV) or rCDV + CAV-2 + CPV ± CPiV Parenteral (SQ)	First dose at or before admission to the shelter. Start as early as 4 wk of age. Repeat every 2–3 wk until 18–20 wk of age[a]	1 dose at or before admission to the shelter. Second dose 2–3 wk later	MLV CPV vaccines have been demonstrated to protect against CPV-2a, -2b, and -2c. rCDV and MLV CDV vaccines provide similar onset of protection when used in animals that lack interfering MDA[17]. Vaccination before 4 wk of age is not recommended because of the immaturity of young puppies' immune system and a possibility that MLV vaccines could cause harm in such animals. CAV-2-containing vaccines protect against CAV-1 and CAV-2
Bb (live, avirulent) ± CPiV (MLV) ± CAV-2 (MLV) Intranasal	A single dose at or before admission to the shelter. Can be given as early as 3–4 wk of age[b]	A single dose at or before admission to the shelter[c]	Bb vaccines can provide disease-sparing protection and reduce shedding but do not induce sterile immunity. MDA does not interfere significantly with mucosal immunity. Every effort should be made to ensure that these intranasal vaccines are not inadvertently injected subcutaneously. The result can be calamitous, if this mistake is made
Bb (live, avirulent) Oral	A single dose at or before admission to the shelter. Can be given as early as 8 wk of age	A single dose at or before admission to the shelter[c]	MDA does not interfere significantly with mucosal immunity. Less is known about this relatively new product. Duration of immunity and effectiveness when given to very young puppies merits further study[21]. Should only be administered orally
Bb (cellular antigen extract) SQ	A first dose at the time of admission (as early as 8 wk of age) followed by a second dose 2 wk later	2 doses, 2 wk apart	Should not be administered via a mucosal route, will be ineffective
Rabies	A single dose at the time of discharge from the facility, if the animal is over 12 wk of age. Revaccination 1 y later	A single dose at the time of discharge from the facility. Revaccination 1 y later	Authority to administer rabies vaccines should be checked. In many jurisdictions, only a licensed veterinarian is permitted to administer rabies vaccines. If dogs are expected to remain in the facility for many months, vaccination at the time of entry is appropriate

Abbreviations: MDA, maternally derived antibodies; rCDV, recombinant CVD; SQ, subcutaneous.
[a] WSAVA recommends revaccination every 2 weeks until 20 weeks of age.
[b] WSAVA recommends a second dose be given after 6 weeks of age.
[c] WSAVA recommends 2 doses, 2 weeks apart.

Table 3
Recommendations derived by review of American Association of Feline Practitioners,[6] World Small Animal Veterinary Association,[4] and European Advisory Board on Cat Diseases[10] guidelines for vaccination of kittens and cats entering and living in shelters

Vaccine	Kittens ≤16–20 wk	Adults	Comments
FPV, FHV-1, FCV (MLV, SQ)	First dose at or before admission to the shelter. Start as early as 4–6 wk of age. Repeat every 2–3 wk until 16–20 wk of age[a]	1 dose at or before admission to the shelter. A second dose 2–3 wk later	The second dose administered to cats is to protect adequately against FHV-1 and FCV. A single dose will protect against FPV. MLV vaccines are generally recommended. They may break through MDA more effectively than inactivated vaccines and provide protection soon after vaccination[20]. MLV vaccines may cause cerebellar hypoplasia if given to kittens younger than 4 wk of age[22]. If fully vaccinated cats in the shelter develop FCV-related disease, benefit may be gained by changing to a vaccine that contains a different FCV strain[23]
FHV-1, FCV (MLV, intranasal) + MLV FPV (SQ)	First dose at or before admission to the shelter. Start as early as 4–6 wk of age. Repeat every 2–3 wk until 16–20 wk of age[a]	1 dose at or before admission to the shelter. A second dose 2–3 wk later	Intranasal vaccination against FHV-1 and FCV must be accompanied by SQ vaccination against FPV. Rapid protection (4–6 d) may be conferred by intranasal respiratory virus vaccines[24]
FeLV; inactivated, subunit, or recombinant	For cats that will be group housed, a first dose as early as 8 wk of age. Repeat 2–3 wk later	1 dose at or before admission to the shelter. A second dose 3–4 wk later	FeLV is an enveloped, fragile virus. The risk of transmission to individually housed cats is low. Conversely, group-housed cats, especially young cats, are at high risk. Vaccination does not substitute for testing and segregation of uninfected from infected cats
Rabies (inactivated or recombinant)	A single dose at the time of discharge from the facility, if the animal is over 12 wk of age. Revaccination 1 y later	A single dose at the time of discharge from the facility. Revaccination 1 y later	Authority to administer rabies vaccines should be checked. In many jurisdictions, only a licensed veterinarian is permitted to administer rabies vaccines. If cats are expected to remain in the facility for many months, vaccination at the time of entry is appropriate

a WSAVA recommends revaccination every 2 weeks until 20 weeks of age. AAFP recommends vaccination every 3 to 4 weeks until 16 weeks of age.

Use of Vaccines in Pregnant, Immunosuppressed, Injured, and Otherwise Ill Animals in Shelters

MLV vaccines can pose risks to unborn puppies and kittens; however, a standard recommendation is to vaccinate pregnant dogs and cats on entry to the shelter, regardless of this risk.[15] A virulent virus poses a greater risk than vaccinal virus. In many cases, pregnant animals will be neutered before being released from the shelter, neutralizing this risk.

MLV vaccines also pose a potential hazard to severely immunosuppressed animals. Again, unless titer testing can be used to avoid unnecessary vaccination, a standard recommendation is to vaccinate with an MLV vaccine on the basis that benefit is very likely to be greater than risk.

Correct Handling of Vaccines

Handling and storage of vaccines in the shelter situation is crucially important. Refrigerators for vaccine storage must be serviceable and regularly checked. Temperature measuring devices can be affixed to refrigerators to help ensure vaccines are stored properly, according to manufacturers' instructions. It is important to ensure that, not only are vaccines kept sufficiently cool but also that they are not stored in a part of the refrigerator that becomes excessively cold, leading to the possibility of vaccines freezing. Lyophilized vaccines should be reconstituted immediately or shortly (minutes) before injection, not hours ahead of time.

Table 2 provides a summary of recommendations made separately by AAHA and WSAVA for vaccination of puppies and dogs entering and living in shelters. **Table 3** provides similar information from the American Association of Feline Practitioners (AAFP) and WSAVA for kittens and cats.

USE OF VACCINES IN OTHER GROUP SETTINGS

The following are some examples of group settings other than animal shelters:

- Boarding kennels and catteries
- Small breeding facilities
- Dog or cat shows
- Sporting events (agility, racing, herding, and hunting)
- Pet daycare facilities
- Puppy socialization events and training sessions
- Cat cafes
- Off-leash dog parks and busy beaches.

This is certainly not a comprehensive list of canine and feline group settings. Research colonies and large, well-run breeding facilities are, for example, not included. These are likely to have sophisticated vaccination protocols appropriate to their specific needs and are not a focus of this article.

In general, guidelines for optimal vaccination of indoor-outdoor pets are sufficient in most of the settings previously listed. Published guidelines recommend that dogs attending many of these activities should be protected against canine infectious respiratory disease in addition to the core diseases. Cats should have received FHV-1 and FCV vaccination within the previous 12 months. Consideration should be given to whether cats living in cat cafes should also be vaccinated against feline immunodeficiency virus (in countries where that vaccine is still marketed) and FeLV.

Boarding kennels and catteries are encouraged to communicate with local veterinary practitioners to develop science-based vaccination requirements for their customers that are appropriate to the local setting. Core vaccines are mandatory for both dogs and cats. Vaccines intended to protect dogs against canine infectious respiratory disease are highly recommended. If cats will be group-housed with unrelated cats in a boarding cattery, FeLV vaccination is strongly recommended. Cats need to have been vaccinated against FHV-1 and FCV within the previous 12 months before going into the boarding cattery. Guidelines for vaccination of cats in breeding catteries have been published.[10]

Puppy socialization during the critical period (approximately 8–14 weeks of age) is recognized to be remarkably important for the development of confident, socially effective adult dogs (https://avsab.org/wp-content/uploads/2016/08/Puppy_Socialization_Position_Statement_Download_-_10-3-14.pdf). The risk of puppies developing CPV-related disease as a consequence of attending well-managed socialization sessions has been studied and found to be remarkably low.[25]

REFERENCES

1. Neiderud C-J. How urbanization affects the epidemiology of emerging infectious diseases. Infect Ecol Epidemiol 2015;5:27060.
2. Dobson AP, Carper ER. Infectious diseases and human population history - Throughout history the establishment of disease has been a side effect of the growth of civilization. Bioscience 1996;46(2):115–26.
3. Hurley KF, Miller L. Introduction to disease management in animal shelters. In: Miller L, Hurley K, editors. Infectious disease management in animal shelters. Ames (IA): Wiley-Blackwell; 2009. p. 5–16.
4. Day MJ, Horzinek MC, Schultz RD, et al, Vaccination Guidelines Group of the World Small Animal Veterinary Association. WSAVA Guidelines for the vaccination of dogs and cats. J Small Anim Pract 2016;57(1):E1–45.
5. Mostl K, Egberink H, Addie D, et al. Prevention of infectious diseases in cat shelters: ABCD guidelines. J Feline Med Surg 2013;15(7):546–54.
6. Scherk MA, Ford RB, Gaskell RM, et al. 2013 AAFP feline vaccination advisory panel report. J Feline Med Surg 2013;15(9):785–808.
7. Hosie MJ, Addie D, Belak S, et al. Matrix vaccination guidelines: ABCD recommendations for indoor/outdoor cats, rescue shelter cats and breeding catteries. J Feline Med Surg 2013;15(7):540–4.
8. Ford RB, Larson LJ, McClure KD, et al. 2017 AAHA canine vaccination guidelines. J Am Anim Hosp Assoc 2017;53(5):243–51.
9. Sparkes A. Feline vaccination protocols: is a consensus emerging? Schweiz Arch Tierheilkd 2010;152(3):135–40.
10. Hosie MJ, Addie DD, Boucraut-Baralon C, et al. Matrix vaccination guidelines: 2015 ABCD recommendations for indoor/outdoor cats, rescue shelter cats and breeding catteries. J Feline Med Surg 2015;17(7):583–7.
11. Zawistowski S, Morris J. Introduction to animal sheltering. In: Miller L, Zawistowski S, editors. Shelter medicine for veterinarians and staff. 2nd edition. Ames (IA): John Wiley and Sons, Inc; 2013. p. 3–12.
12. Litster A, Nichols J, Volpe A. Prevalence of positive antibody test results for canine parvovirus (CPV) and canine distemper virus (CDV) and response to modified live vaccination against CPV and CDV in dogs entering animal shelters. Vet Microbiol 2012;157(1–2):86–90.
13. Lechner ES, Crawford PC, Levy JK, et al. Prevalence of protective antibody titers for canine distemper virus and canine parvovirus in dogs entering a Florida animal shelter. J Am Vet Med Assoc 2010;236(12):1317–21.

14. DiGangi BA, Levy JK, Griffin B, et al. Prevalence of serum antibody titers against feline panleukopenia virus, feline herpesvirus 1, and feline calicivirus in cats entering a Florida animal shelter. J Am Vet Med Assoc 2012;241(10):1320–5.

15. Larson LJ, Newbury S, Schultz RD. Canine and feline vaccinations and immunology. In: Miller L, Hurley K, editors. Infectious disease management in animal shelters. Ames (IA): Wiley-Blackwell; 2009. p. 61–82.

16. Gingrich E, Lappin M. Practical overview of common infectious disease agents. In: Miller L, Zawistowski S, editors. Shelter medicine for veterinarians and staff. 2nd edition. Ames (IA): Wiley-Blackwell; 2013. p. 297–328.

17. Larson LJ, Schultz RD. Effect of vaccination with recombinant canine distemper virus vaccine immediately before exposure under shelter-like conditions. Vet Ther 2006;7(2):113–8.

18. Ellis JA. How well do vaccines for *Bordetella bronchiseptica* work in dogs? A critical review of the literature 1977-2014. Vet J 2015;204(1):5–16.

19. Schultz RD. Duration of immunity for canine and feline vaccines: a review. Vet Microbiol 2006;117(1):75–9.

20. Digangi BA, Levy JK, Griffin B, et al. Effects of maternally-derived antibodies on serologic responses to vaccination in kittens. J Feline Med Surg 2012;14(2):118–23.

21. Ellis JA, Gow SP, Waldner CL, et al. Comparative efficacy of intranasal and oral vaccines against *Bordetella bronchiseptica* in dogs. Vet J 2016;212:71–7.

22. Aeffner F, Ulrich R, Schulze-Ruckamp L, et al. Cerebellar hypoplasia in three sibling cats after intrauterine or early postnatal parvovirus infection. Dtsch Tierarztl Wochenschr 2006;113(11):403–6.

23. Radford AD, Addie D, Belak S, et al. Feline calicivirus infection ABCD guidelines on prevention and management. J Feline Med Surg 2009;11(7):556–64.

24. Lappin MR, Sebring RW, Porter M, et al. Effects of a single dose of an intranasal feline herpesvirus 1, calicivirus, and panleukopenia vaccine on clinical signs and virus shedding after challenge with virulent feline herpesvirus 1. J Feline Med Surg 2006;8(3):158–63.

25. Stepita ME, Bain MJ, Kass PH. Frequency of CPV infection in vaccinated puppies that attended puppy socialization classes. J Am Anim Hosp Assoc 2013;49(2):95–100.

Prevention of Feline Injection-Site Sarcomas

Is There a Scientific Foundation for Vaccine Recommendations at This Time?

Philip H. Kass, DVM, MPVM, MS, PhD

KEYWORDS

- Injection-site sarcoma • Vaccines • Adverse reactions • Cat

KEY POINTS

- Authority figures have made vaccine recommendations to reduce the incidence of feline injection-site sarcomas.
- The evidence supporting these vaccine recommendations is surprisingly weak.
- Until additional research is performed, there is little evidence supporting the recommendation that use of certain vaccines will prevent sarcoma formation.

Over 25 years have passed since the initial report of vaccine-site sarcomas (FISS) appeared in the veterinary medical literature.[1] Almost from the point of recognition of these iatrogenic tumors, the veterinary medical profession and its allied professional communities have valiantly struggled to promulgate recommendations to mitigate, if not eliminate, the risks associated with vaccinations. Examples of such recommendations have included avoidance of multidose vaccine vials, distributing vaccines over different parts of the body, using vaccines less likely to induce local inflammation, restricting vaccines to cats with potential exposure to other animals with communicable diseases, and even not vaccinating at all.

One article, "Feline Injection-site sarcoma: ABCD guidelines on prevention and management"[2] encapsulates considerable thought to date, and perhaps even mainstream credence on strategies for treating and preventing these iatrogenic tumors, products of the veterinary medical profession's well-intentioned and largely successful attempt to eliminate the incidence of rabies and, to a lesser extent, other mostly species-specific infectious diseases in domestic cat populations. Given the widespread market penetration of vaccines in the United States, Canada, and many

Disclosure Statement: The author has nothing to disclose.
Department of Population Health and Reproduction, School of Veterinary Medicine, University of California, 1089 Veterinary Medicine Drive, Davis, CA 95616, USA
E-mail address: phkass@ucdavis.edu

countries of Europe, together with the large number of owned cats, there are now more than 20 years of experience managing afflicted patients, providing a plethora of information about current standards of practice as well as emerging state-of-the-art therapies. The veterinary medical professional manifestly benefits from such reflection, as do owners and their feline companions.

I am less sanguine, however, that these authors' recommendations for prevention share the same evidence-based scientific standing that their management recommendations have. For there to be standing to justify recommendations there must be foundation. For there to be foundation there must be evidence; for there to be evidence there must be research. The latter presents in many forms, and I have become increasingly concerned that the findings from preliminary or tenuous research have, over time, taken on a quasi-mythical standing through a disciplinary support network that places more weight on belief than on the weight of the evidence itself. Opinion is, of course, the natural evolution of the assimilation of information, and is the provenance of assertions by decision makers occupying positions of leadership, influence, and change. In the proper setting, and in the appropriate context, such expressions contribute to a healthy exchange and dialogue (eg, the Vaccine-Associated Feline Sarcoma Task Force).[3] For an article focusing on prevention of this disease in a peer-reviewed scientific journal, far more circumspection is not only warranted, but arguably essential. In this article, I hope to underscore this contention by illustrating that not only do I judge that such recommendations are premature (although not necessarily incorrect), but that others absorbing the same body of evidence could be impelled to reach entirely different conclusions.

The key statement in that article, and hence the most provocative, is the following from the abstract: "Non-adjuvanted, modified-live or recombinant vaccines should be selected in preference to adjuvanted vaccines." This is manifestly similar to a principle expressed in the World Small Animal Veterinary Association's (WSAVA) Guidelines for the Vaccination of Dog and Cats[4]: "Non-adjuvanted vaccines should be administered to cats wherever possible." Indeed, the WSAVA[4] and Hartmann and colleagues[2] articles share authors in common. However, these prescriptions go well beyond the recommendations of the 2013 American Association of Feline Practitioners Advisory Panel Report, which judiciously exercised considerably more restraint in writing: "Overall, however, the Advisory Panel concluded that, at the current time, there is insufficient information to make definitive recommendations to use particular vaccine types to reduce the risk of FISS [feline injection-site sarcomas]."[5]

What is the evidence to support the Hartmann and colleagues[2] recommendation, as indicated in the abstract and on page 611: "Vaccines without adjuvants should be used rather than adjuvant-containing vaccines, which means that MLV or recombinant vaccines (eg, canarypox-vectored vaccine) without adjuvant are preferred over inactivated vaccines with adjuvants?" The section "Recommendations for reducing inflammatory reactions" (pages 610–611) provides some guidance. Three articles cited found that recombinant canarypox-vectored vaccines caused less inflammation when injected into rats and cats.[6–8]

The use of such experimental studies to measure postvaccinal tissue inflammation is enigmatic and can be faulted on several grounds. Using rodents as models of adjuvant-induced inflammation or carcinogenesis in the cat remains notional, and its validity has previously been called into question.[9] Given the near-certain differences between species in immunologic and tissue-based responses to vaccine adjuvants, it should be difficult to ascribe more than a passing interest in these results. As for the use of cats in experimental studies, the goal should not be to measure relative inflammatory responses, which would inevitably be expected under different vaccine formulations, but rather to estimate neoplastic incidence. None of these experimental studies, however, had anything close to the statistical power necessary to detect differences in vaccine risk. Suppose, for example, that the incidence of sarcomas following vaccination is 5 cases in 10,000 cat-doses, and the incidence in the absence of vaccines is 1 case in 10,000 cat-doses (ie, the relative risk is 5). A prospective 2-armed randomized study analyzed with a 2-sided Pearson's chi-square test, with equal allocation between arms and Type I and Type II error proportions of 5%, would require almost 100,000 cats. In contrast, the experimental studies in rats and cats cited previously had sample sizes in the double-digits.

Although they employed different methods to arrive at their respective conclusions, the experimental studies, not unexpectedly, shared a key critical feature: none of the study subjects developed injection site sarcomas. Although their findings may have implications for the study of postvaccinal inflammatory responses, they fail to provide a rational basis for making causal inferences about vaccine propensity to induce tumorigenesis. Such a causal connection between postvaccinal inflammation and tumorigenesis remains to this day one entirely of conjecture, speculation, and hypothesis, and until that connection can be firmly established, such articles may be useful in understanding vaccine-specific inflammation, but have unproven and hence questionable value in understanding vaccine formulation-specific risk of sarcoma development. They and others (eg, the vaccine manufacturer-funded experimental Grosenbaugh and colleagues[10] study) emphatically do not rise to the level of research upon which policy supported by science about reducing the incidence of injection-site sarcomas should be promulgated and distributed.

Nevertheless, this has not prevented several authors from doing exactly that,[11–14] a practice that at this time I consider to be imprudent. Of considerable concern is that these articles include unpublished data, personal communications, citations of review articles, reliance on science by authority, or engagement in associational speculation. It is also sometimes the case that authors have financial ties, as collaborators, consultants, or employees, to the very industries that are impacted by their recommendations. It must be incumbent on all authors (and presenters) in the field of FISS to fully disclose such relationships to their readers (and audiences) to further transparency and scientific integrity.

The final article the authors invoked to support their recommendation is from my own research group at the University of California, Davis.[15] And although this study did include cats with injection-site sarcomas, and indeed found supportive evidence for differential tumorigenic propensity between vaccine types, I would firmly contend that it alone (discounting the previously mentioned articles about inflammation but not sarcomas) remains insufficient to this day to be the basis for the recommendations in Hartmann and colleagues[2] In fact, we attempted to temper our findings within the article itself by citing the study's shortcomings that could pose a threat to validity:

A low response rate from veterinarians, which could have been differential with respect to the types of vaccines administered

A small sample size, which makes a single study far more susceptible to biased and imprecise estimates

Missing data

The use of multiple vaccines at the same site either at one or multiple times

The tendency to report a single number or conclusion from a single study is unfortunately all too common, and I have witnessed individual odds ratios (ORs) from this study presented outside of their proper statistical context. For example, Srivastav and colleagues[15] reported that "... there was evidence of a significantly lower frequency of use of recombinant rabies vaccines in case cats than controls. Using cats with nonvaccine site sarcomas as controls, in years 1, 2, and 3, the ORs were 0.1 (95% CI, 0.0–0.7; P = .014), 0.1 (95% CI, 0.0–0.4; P = .001), and 0.1 (95% CI, 0.0–0.6; P = .005), respectively." At a recent international meeting, I heard these findings communicated as: the odds of cases receiving a nonrecombinant vaccine was tenfold greater than receiving a recombinant vaccine (ie, 1/0.1 = 10). Although literally correct in an algebraic sense, such statements entirely ignore a key purpose of statistical inference in the first place: the analysis of variance. Focusing solely on point estimates fails to convey important information (eg, an OR of 10 from a sample size of 50 should naturally be given far less credibility than an odds ratio of 10 from a sample size of 500). A more recent presentation at least pointed out that the CI around the communicated value of 10 would have been (using, for example, the year 2 value) 2.5 to infinity.[16] But the real story about the quantitative relationship between vaccine type and sarcoma incidence, which from this article is profoundly imprecise, is how little we still really understand even after this study's publication. Moreover, it is often unappreciated that the P-values associated with such tests are only correct insofar as the assumptions underlying them are accurate, including the absence of bias, under the probability distribution model utilized in the analysis. In other words, if any of the biases noted previously were present, then regardless of the statistical significance, the P-values would be incorrect, as would the point estimates (ORs) and CIs. It is a scientific disservice to recapitulate potentially headline-grabbing findings from articles without concomitantly and fully assessing and disclosing those features that could adversely impact study accuracy. Far too often excessive credence is placed on statistical significance, and far too little weight on the myriad subtleties of observational study design and analysis that can lead to invalid inferences:

Errors of comparisons (confounding bias)
Errors in selection of study subjects (selection bias)
Errors in (often historical) measurements (information bias)
Errors in statistical modeling (specification bias)

In the case of the Srivastav and colleagues article,[15] such threats to validity could include (but are not limited to):

The low veterinarian participation rate (eg, participation could be related to veterinarian preference for vaccine type)
Diagnostic work-up being related to type of vaccine administered
Missing data that could have been related to type of vaccine administered

I contend that the authors' avidity for their prevention recommendations[2] exceeds the weight of foundational scientific evidence to support them at this time. Although they apparently consider them to be accurate, and they may be correct, the insertion of such recommendations into such an authoritative report strikes me as premature, fails to convey the paucity of evidence supporting them, and omits a critical analysis of research upon which they are based. It is evocative of the admonitions of author/journalist Christopher Hitchens: "Forgotten were the elementary rules of logic, that extraordinary claims require extraordinary evidence and that what can be asserted without evidence can also be dismissed without evidence."[17] A similar forewarning about the shortcomings of published research was forcefully made by Ioannides,[18] who wrote: "Several methodologists have pointed out that the high rate of nonreplication (lack of confirmation) of research discoveries is a consequence of the convenient, yet ill-founded strategy of claiming conclusive research findings solely based on a single study assessed by formal statistical significance, typically for a *P*-value less than 0.05." All too often, human medicine has been forced to disavow widely disseminated public health recommendations founded on nonexperimental studies when later, more robust evidence failed to support their establishment.[19] I only hope that history does not repeat itself here.

REFERENCES

1. Hendrick MJ, Goldschmidt MH. Do injection site reactions induce fibrosarcomas in cats? J Am Vet Med Assoc 1991;199:968.
2. Hartmann K, Day MJ, Thiry E, et al. Feline injection-site sarcoma: ABCD guidelines on prevention and management. J Feline Med Surg 2015;17:606–13.
3. Vaccine-Associated Feline Sarcoma Task Force. The current understanding and management of vaccine-associated sarcomas in cats. J Am Vet Med Assoc 2005;226:1821–42.
4. Day MJ, Horzinek MC, Schultz RD, et al. WSAVA guidelines for the vaccination of dogs and cats. J Small Anim Pract 2016;57:E1–45.
5. Scherk MA, Ford RB, Gaskell M, et al. 2013 AAFP feline vaccination advisory panel report. J Feline Med Surg 2013;15:785–808.
6. Devauchelle P, Magnol JP. Dynamique de la réaction inflammatoire induite chez le chat par l'administration sous-cutanée d'un vaccine non adjuvé. In: Proc Conférence Nationale des Vétérinaires Spécialistes en Petits Animaux (CNVSPA) Congress. Lille (France), November 23–25, 2001.
7. Macy DW, Chretin J. Local postvaccinal reactions of a recombinant rabies vaccine. Vet Forum 1999;16:44–9.
8. Day MJ, Schoon HA, Magnol JP, et al. A kinetic study of histopathological changes in the subcutis of cats injected with non-adjuvanted and adjuvanted multi-component vaccines. Vaccine 2007;25:4073–84.
9. Spickler AR, Roth JA. Adjuvants in veterinary vaccines: modes of action and adverse effects. J Vet Intern Med 2003;17:273–81.
10. Grosenbaugh DA, Leard T, Pardo MC, et al. Comparison of the safety and efficacy of a recombinant feline leukemia virus (FeLV) vaccine delivered transdermally and an inactivated FeLV vaccine delivered subcutaneously. Vet Ther 2004;5:258–62.
11. Macy DW. Current understanding of vaccination site-associated sarcomas in the cat. J Feline Med Surg 1999;1:15–21.
12. Macy DW. Feline vaccine-associated sarcomas: progress? Anim Health Res Rev 2004;5:287–9.
13. Hauck M. Feline injection site sarcomas. Vet Clin North Am Small Anim Pract 2003;33:553–71.
14. Horzinek MC, Thiry E. Vaccines and vaccination: the principles and the polemics. J Feline Med Surg 2009;11:530–7.
15. Srivastav A, Kass PH, McGill LD, et al. Comparative vaccine-specific and other injectable-specific risks of injection-site sarcomas in cats. J Am Vet Med Assoc 2012;241:595–602.
16. Wolf A. Feline vaccination - 2017. Colorado Veterinary Medical Association. Available at: https://www.google.com/url?sa=t&rct=j&q=&esrc=s&source=web&cd=1&ved=0ahUKEwiah5OWwYXWAhWJ0FQKHZGPD50QFggmMAA&url=http%3A%2F%2Fcolovma.org%2Fwp-content%2Fuploads%2Fsites%2F4%2F2017%2F02%2FAlice-Wolf-DVM.pdf&usg=AFQjCNFPemgefHzN3OJocmZLw2hA8002pQ. Accessed September 12, 2017.

17. Hitchens C. Mommie dearest. Slate. 2003. Available at: http://www.slate.com/articles/news_and_politics/fighting_words/2003/10/mommie_dearest.html. Accessed September 12, 2017.
18. Ioannidis JPA. Why most published research findings are false. PLoS Med 2005; 2(8):e124.
19. Taubes G. Do we really know what makes us healthy? The New York Times Magazine. 2007. Available at: http://www.nytimes.com/2007/09/16/magazine/16epidemiology-t.html?_r=0. Accessed September 12, 2017.

The Microbiota Regulates Immunity and Immunologic Diseases in Dogs and Cats

Ian R. Tizard, BVMS, PhD, DSc, ACVM*, Sydney W. Jones, BS

KEYWORDS

- Microbiota • Dysbiosis • Hygiene hypothesis • Atopic dermatitis • Allergies
- Autoimmunity

KEY POINTS

- It is now possible, by the use of modern sequencing techniques, to determine the composition of the microbiota on body surfaces, especially the skin and gastrointestinal tract.
- The microbiota influences the development and functions of the immune system.
- In healthy animals, the microbiota and the immune system maintain a balance so that excessive immune and inflammatory responses are avoided.
- Disturbances in the composition of the microbiota (dysbiosis) permit the development of inflammatory and allergic diseases (the hygiene hypothesis).
- Important diseases triggered in dogs and cats by dysbiosis include respiratory allergies, atopic dermatitis, and inflammatory bowel disease.

Animals are obliged to develop a relationship with the microbes that live on their surfaces. The enormous and diverse population of microorganisms living on the skin and within the respiratory and digestive tracts directly influences the development, regulation, and function of the immune system. Conversely, the immune system regulates the composition and behavior of these microbial populations. Immune responses are therefore profoundly influenced by the microbiota.

Body surfaces constitute stable, nutrient-rich ecosystems where microbes thrive. As a result, they are densely populated by bacteria, archea, fungi, and viruses, collectively termed the microbiota. It is estimated that in an animal body at least half of all the cells are microbial. These microbes release a complex mixture of metabolites, vitamins, and nutrients that signal to the host's immune system and influence the immune

The authors have nothing to disclose.
Department of Veterinary Pathobiology, College of Veterinary Medicine, Texas A&M University, MS#4467, College Station, TX 77843, USA
* Corresponding author.
E-mail address: itizard@cvm.tamu.edu

Vet Clin Small Anim 48 (2018) 307–322
https://doi.org/10.1016/j.cvsm.2017.10.008

vetsmall.theclinics.com

system development, function, and behavior.[1] This is reflected in profound effects on the development of immunologic and allergic diseases. These microbial effects must be considered while treating such complex diseases and they provide possible routes to new innovative treatments.

The body's surface defenses are faced with the task of coexisting with the microbiota while simultaneously preventing any invasion of pathogens through breaks in the epithelial barriers. Nutrients and microbial metabolites are continually released into the body by the microbiota where they influence immune cell and inflammatory functions. These products, detected by the cells of the immune system, ensure that the immune system is prepared to respond promptly to microbial invasion.[2] In fact, the body's response to the microbiota involves 2 opposing processes. Stimulation by microbial products serves to activate the immune system. However, to ensure that inflammation and other immune processes are not excessive, this stimulatory response must be counterbalanced by regulatory processes.

For many years, it was believed that the role of the immune system was simply to ensure exclusion of all invading microbes by distinguishing between self and not-self and eliminating foreign antigens. It is now known, however, that the immune system must also determine the degree and nature of the threat posed by the microbes it encounters and adjust its responses accordingly. It must tolerate the microbiota and food antigens while simultaneously be highly responsive to invading pathogens. It must decide, when necessary, whether to mount a cell-mediated or an antibody-mediated response. This discrimination is determined both by how the antigens are processed and by signals from the microbiota. The presence of the microbiota must either be tolerated or ignored if an animal is to remain healthy. An animal cannot afford to act aggressively toward its own microbiota. The presence of all these bacterial products has the potential to trigger massive acute inflammation; however, this inflammation must not happen unless absolutely required to defend the body.

Therefore, in a normal, healthy animal, 2 opposing responses are in balance. The body, although not responding aggressively to the microbiota, must be prepared to respond rapidly and effectively at any time. The body must refrain from overresponding aggressively to the microbiota while being ready to respond rapidly and effectively when necessary.

If this equilibrium between the proinflammatory and antiinflammatory processes is disturbed, this will be reflected in changes in the level of activation of the immune and inflammatory systems.

HOW THE MICROBIOTA IS ANALYZED

The existence of the microbiota has been known since the invention of the microscope. Its importance, however, has been generally underappreciated until recently. Advances in technology have allowed for a deeper understanding of the complex ecosystem of the microbiome and its interactions with the host immune system.

In the past, intestinal bacteria were identified by growing them in culture; however, this only allowed a small proportion of the highly diverse microbial ecosystem to be identified. The anaerobic nature and restricted cultural conditions of most gut bacteria in cats and dogs, as well as limited knowledge of appropriate media for many bacterial species, prevent culturing them.[3–6] However, prokaryotes can now be identified and classified within complex mixtures by sequencing their specific DNA. As a result, much of the characterization of the gastrointestinal microbiota has focused on the bacterial composition. Although commensal archaea, fungi, and viruses reside in the gut, their role in the health and disease of the host, although clearly important, remains poorly understood.[7–9]

There are many molecular tools that can be used to characterize the microbiota. This analysis first requires acquisition of an appropriate intestinal sample (feces, luminal content, or biopsy; swab or scrape in cases of postmortem sample collection) from which DNA or RNA can be extracted. The sample DNA is extracted, isolated, and purified. This DNA can then be identified by amplifying specific genes using universal primers, and quantified using quantitative real-time polymerase chain reaction (qPCR) and fluorescent in situ hybridization (FISH).[7]

For phylogenetic identification, the 16S ribosomal RNA (rRNA) gene, which encodes the small subunit of rRNA and is thus present in all bacteria, is often targeted.[6,7,9] The 16S rRNA gene is found only in prokaryotes and, although highly conserved within a bacterial species, it contains hypervariable regions with specific sequences that can be used to identify the bacterial species.[7] These 16S rRNA genes are sequenced using primer sets that amplify 1 of their hypervariable regions. A next-generation sequencing platform, such as the Illumina platform or 454-pyrosequencing, can be used to produce reads of about 75 to 500 base pairs. This is only a small portion of the 16S rRNA gene which, in total, contains approximately 1500 base pairs. Using platforms such as these is more cost-effective than complete genome sequencing and still permits 1 or 2 specific hypervariable regions to be assembled. Other methods of sequencing include shotgun metagenomics and transcriptomics, which through new high-throughput sequencing platforms permits sequencing of the total genomic DNA or mRNA without previously amplifying specific genes.[6,7,9] These methods permit determination of a core microbiome, defined as the number and identity of bacteria that are shared among different individuals, and identification of a functional profile of the microbiome.[6,7,9] Metabolomics using mass spectrometry to examine the metabolites produced by bacteria can be used to analyze changes in biochemical pathways of the host caused by dysbiosis.[6,7,9] Molecular fingerprinting produces a representation of the bacterial community through separation of a mixture of polymerase chain reaction (PCR) amplicons generated by universal primers. Different techniques can be used in molecular fingerprinting, including denaturing gradient gel electrophoresis (DGGE) and temperature gradient gel electrophoresis (TGGE), and terminal restriction fragment length polymorphism.[6] Although these techniques are inexpensive and can be performed rapidly, DGGE and TGGE only allow changes in the predominant bacterial groups to be examined. Quantification of bacterial groups can be done using qPCR and FISH.[6]

Following sequencing, bioinformatics analysis of the raw DNA data can be performed. The bacterial population is compared with a comprehensive database of known 16S rRNA genes, permitting classification and identification of the microbes present. Duplicates are removed, as are reads that indicate plant material, eukaryotes, and archaea, which suggest the presence of contaminants such as food or host genomic material. The remaining sequences can then be assigned into groups known as operational taxonomic units, which refer to clusters of unknown organisms that are grouped by similarity of their DNA sequence (eg, the 16S rRNA marker gene). Several statistical methods and programs are available to analyze the data obtained. Many of the measures used in microbiome analyses are also commonly used in ecology. For example, evaluation of the bacterial species richness and diversity can be accomplished by determining the alpha and beta diversity (alpha diversity is a measure of diversity within samples, whereas beta diversity measures diversity between samples), which are commonly used in population studies in ecology. The need to analyze microbial diversity using ecological techniques reinforces the idea that the micro-biome is a complex ecosystem composed of a diverse array of metabolically active organisms.

THE NORMAL MICROBIOTA

The development of the immune system in newborn puppies and kittens is driven by the organisms that colonize the skin and the gastrointestinal and respiratory tracts. These early-life microbial exposures determine how the immune system develops because germ-free mammals fail to develop their mucosal lymphoid tissues. The microbiota generates a complex mixture of microbial-associated molecular patterns that act through enterocyte toll-like receptors (TLRs) to promote the functional devel-opment of the immune system.[10] The intestinal and skin microbiota also contributes to this process as newborns suckle and are groomed by the mother.[11]

The Skin

Normal skin harbors trillions of microorganisms on keratinocytes and within seba-ceous glands and hair follicles.[12] It has been estimated that up to a billion bacteria may live on a square centimeter of human skin. Given the sheltering effects of hairs or feathers, it is likely that the skin microbiota in domestic animals is even more com-plex. The skin microbiota of dogs varies greatly between individuals and different skin sites. For example, there is higher microbial diversity in haired skin compared with mucocutaneous junctions. The precise composition of the skin microbiota thus de-pends on location (hairy, wooly, or bald skin; back vs skin in the axilla, groin, or ear) and the presence of disease such as seborrhea or atopic dermatitis (AD). Grooming activities have some impact on these microbial populations but their significance is unclear. The highest microbial diversity on dogs was found in the axilla and the dorsum of the nose. On average about 300 different bacterial species were identified on the dorsal canine nose.[13] Large populations of Proteobacteria and Oxalobacteraceae pre-dominate. The feline skin microbiota is also highly diverse. The most common phyla are Proteobacteria, followed by Bacteroidetes, Firmicutes, Actinobacteria, and Fuso-bacteria. Major changes in abundance are also observed at different skin sites.[14,15]

In mice, the skin microbiota influences local inflammatory and T-cell responses. The microbiota controls the balance between effector and regulatory T (Treg) cells within skin tissue. They influence keratinocyte production of interleukin (IL)-1 and its effects on epidermal dendritic cells and thus control local T-cell responses.[16,17] Skin bacteria may activate antigen-specific T cells across the intact epithelium. However, the pres-ence of Treg cells in neonatal skin mediates tolerance to skin commensal bacteria at a time when the skin is establishing its microbiota.

The Respiratory Tract

Like all body surfaces, the upper respiratory tract houses a dense and complex micro-biota. It has been calculated that a human inhales 10^5 organisms per day just breath-ing outdoor air. Many nasal bacteria are also found on the skin, whereas others are common environmental bacteria. Deeper in the airways, in the lower respiratory tract, Neisseria and gram-negative cocci are common.[18] The lung is not sterile. Healthy lungs harbor a microbiota closely related to but much less dense than in the upper res-piratory tract. The bronchi contain about 2000 bacterial genomes per 1 cm^2. Lung tis-sues contain between 10 and 100 bacterial cells per 1000 lung cells. These include aerobes and anaerobes and, like other surfaces, they differ greatly between individ-uals. The predominant phyla are Firmicutes with lesser numbers of Proteobacteria and Actinobacteria. The organisms found within the mucous layer include not only bacteria but also fungi (yeasts) and viruses such as bacteriophages.[19]

The Genitourinary System

In adult female animals, lactobacilli and other lactic acid-producing bacteria dominate the healthy cervicovaginal microbiota. The vagina is also lined by squamous epithelial cells rich in glycogen. When these epithelial cells desquamate, the glycogen provides a substrate for the lactobacilli that, in turn, produce large quantities of lactic acid. This reduces the pH to a level that protects the vagina against invasion by many pathogenic bacteria and yeasts. Glycogen storage in the vaginal epithelial cells is stimulated by estrogens and thus occurs only in sexually mature animals.

The Gastrointestinal Tract

The gastrointestinal tract contains an incredibly complex mixture of bacteria, archea, fungi, and viruses. The most obvious of these are trillions of bacteria belonging to hundreds of different species. In mammals, they are dominated by members of 2 phyla: the Firmicutes and the Bacteroidetes, with lesser numbers of Actinobacteria and Proteobacteria, and many minor phyla such as the Fusobacteria and the Verrucomicrobia. Mammals possess about 20,000 protein-encoding genes, whereas their microbiota may collectively possess about 10 million. These diverse genomes enhance an animal's metabolic potential. They increase its ability to extract energy from plant structural carbohydrates and to obtain essential vitamins. Because of the microbiota, animals can use food sources that would otherwise be unavailable. For example, mice with a conventional microbiota need to eat 30% fewer calories than so-called germ-free mice to maintain their body weight.

Dogs

The dog is more omnivorous than the cat and can digest and absorb a significant amount of carbohydrates. However, it does not depend on microbial fermentation as a major energy source. Nevertheless, a balanced microbiota is essential for canine gastrointestinal health. Each individual dog's intestinal microbiota is unique and its composition is determined by management, diet, genetics, antibiotic exposure, and environmental factors. The composition of the microbiota also changes along the gastrointestinal tract under the influence of nutrient availability and the local microenvironment.[4]

The canine stomach has a microbiome dominated by *Helicobacter* spp. Bacterial counts in the canine duodenum are in a range from 10^2 to 10^9 per gram of content. In the colon, the count ranges from 10^9 to 10^{11} colony forming units per gram. The predominant intestinal phyla include the Firmicutes (48%), Bacteroidetes (12%), Proteobacteria (23%), Fusobacteria (17%), and Actinobacteria (1%).[20] Clostridiales predominate in the duodenum and jejunum. Fusobacteriales and Bacteroidetes are most abundant in the ileum and colon. Variations result from differences in breed, diet, and age. The Firmicutes consist of mainly gram-positive bacteria, many of which are spore-forming. Important members include Clostridia that may be beneficial or pathogenic. They also include potentially pathogenic Streptococci and Staphylococci. The Actinobacteria are also gram-positive bacteria but with a different G + C content than the Firmicutes. The Bacteroidetes are gram-negative bacteria that ferment indigestible plant carbohydrates to produce short-chain fatty acids (SCFAs). The Proteobacteria include the gram-negative enterobacteria such as *Escherichia coli* and Klebsiella.

Cats

The intestinal microbiota of the cat, like that of the dog, has evolved with a carnivorous diet. As a result, the cat does not depend on the microbiota to maintain an energy balance. As obligate carnivores, domestic cats rely on a high protein diet. Their predominant phyla include Firmicutes (68%), Proteobacteria (14%), Bacteroidetes (10%), Fusobacteria (5%), and Actinobacteria (4%).[20]

THE MICROBIOTA AND THE IMMUNE SYSTEM
Intestinal Protection

The microbiota protects the body against invasion by pathogens by competing for essential metabolites and nutrients, and by inducing intestinal immune responses. By occupying and exploiting the intestinal niche, commensal bacteria block subsequent colonization by pathogenic bacteria.[21] The microbiota also modifies the intestinal environment by maintaining a low pH and oxygen tension. There is more immune system activity in the intestine than in all other lymphoid tissues combined. It has been estimated that more than 80% of the body's activated B cells are found in the intestine. Their function is to defend against possible invasion by the microbiota. However, the key to successful accommodation with the intestinal microbiota also depends on the body's ability to regulate inflammation in the gut wall.[21,22] This is achieved by maintaining a balance between proinflammatory Th17 cells and antiinflammatory Treg cells.

By studying the changes in the immune system in mice colonized by a single species of bacterium, it has been demonstrated that many different bacteria affect immune function. Many bacterial species have similar, overlapping, or even opposite functions. The enormous diversity and redundancy of the microbiota exerts a complex collective effect on the immune system.[23] Some are potent stimulators of Th17 cells, whereas about a quarter of the bacteria studied stimulate Treg cells. Other bacteria affect innate lymphoid cells (ILCs) and dendritic cells.

Development of Lymphoid Organs

It has long been possible to derive animals by cesarean surgery and raise them within sealed chambers in such a way that they are free of microbes. Compared with conventionally raised animals, these germ-free animals have fewer and smaller Peyer's patches, smaller mesenteric lymph nodes, and fewer CD4[+] T cells in the lamina propria of the gut wall.[24] They also have fewer intraepithelial T lymphocytes (IELs) within their intestinal epithelium. These IELs have reduced expression of TLRs and major histocompatibility complex (MHC) class II molecules, as well as reduced cytotoxicity. Germ-free mice have fewer CD4[+] T cells in the spleen, and fewer and smaller germinal centers, as a result of reduced B-cell numbers. Their production of macrophages and neutrophils is impaired, and their immunoglobulin levels are only about 2% of normal. If exposed abruptly to the external environment, these animals are vulnerable to bacterial invasion.

Mammals have evolved several strategies to generate a diverse antibody repertoire. Thus cattle, sheep, pigs, and rabbits undertake an initial burst of B-cell proliferation with limited diversification in utero. These newly produced cells then migrate to the gut-associated lymphoid tissues where they expand both their numbers and their diversity. This microbial driven B-cell diversification and IgA production depends on the presence of certain bacteria within the microbiota.[25] For example, a combination of *Bacteroides fragilis* and *Bacillus subtilis* can induce B-cell development and VDJ diversification in germ-free rabbits. Neither species alone has this effect, suggesting that 2 signals are needed.[26,27] It is thought that microbial molecules trigger these B-cell responses by binding to their TLRs and activating nuclear factor kappa B (NF-κB) pathways. Alternatively, soluble bacterial superantigens might trigger a polyclonal B-cell response and drive the process by preferentially stimulating the production of B cells expressing certain Vh regions.

Signals from the Microbiota to the Body

Bacteria, be they on the skin, respiratory tract, genital tract, or intestine, communicate directly and effectively with their host's immune system through metabolites and nutrients (**Fig. 1**). Indeed, this interaction is essential to the proper functioning of the innate and adaptive immune responses.[28] Alterations or imbalances in the microbiota therefore have profound effects on immune functions.[29] The proper interaction between the immune system and the microbiota is required for optimal animal health.

Dietary plant fibers contain complex carbohydrates. When digested by Clostridia in the cecum and colon, these carbohydrates generate SCFAs, such as butyrate, propionate, and acetate, which suppress macrophages and promote production of Treg cells. As a result, high-fiber diets play a key role in regulating intestinal inflammation.

Among the intestinal microbiota, some bacteria play a key role in regulating immune responses. For example, Clostridia clusters IV, XIVa, and XVIII specifically induce Treg cells by enterocytes and thus suppress inflammation. The presence of these Clostridial clusters in the colon also results in an increase in the numbers of Treg cells in distant tissues such as the spleen and lung, and they play a role in inhibiting allergic responses.[30] Thus T cells educated by commensal bacteria emigrate from the gut to remote tissues and determine the body's T-cell balance.

Enterocytes interact with the intestinal microbiota in a multitude of ways.[31] They produce peptides that kill or inactivate bacteria and, as a result, shape its composition. They block access of intact antigens to the lamina propria, secrete, and respond to regulatory cytokines and display antigens to dendritic cells. They are vital in ensuring that a balance exists between inflammation and tolerance of the microbiota.[31] Within the epithelium and the underlying lamina propria are IELs that, on appropriate stimulation by microbiota-induced IL-1 or IL-23, can regulate their differentiation into effector or regulatory cells. By preventing microbial invasion, enterocytes also prevent

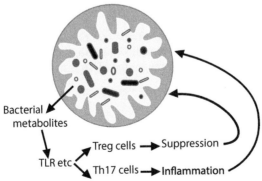

Fig. 1. Microbial products and nutrients pass through the intestinal wall and regulate the development and activities of the immune system by maintaining a balance between immunosuppressive Treg cells and proinflammatory Th17 cells. If the microbiota composition changes and dysbiosis results, this balance may be disrupted and animals may become predisposed to developing inflammatory and allergic diseases.

the development of inflammation within the intestinal wall [32]. Antimicrobial peptides within the inner mucous layer keep most of the microbiota from contacting the enterocytes and thus ensure that the microbiota is confined to the intestinal lumen. They not only protect the host from microbial invasion but also from the potentially harmful inflammatory response that would occur if excessive microbial products are absorbed into the body.

Group 3 ILC also regulate the interactions between the microbiota and its host.[32–34] They produce IL-17 and IL-22 that attract neutrophils and promote the production of antimicrobial peptides in the small intestine. ILC3 cells also activate B cells and induce IgA production.[35]

Although gut microbes are separated by the inner mucous layer and glycocalyx from direct contact with enterocytes, intestinal dendritic cells can extend their dendrites into the intestinal lumen and sample the microbiota. These bacteria may persist within the dendritic cells for several days while they are transported into the mucosa and mesenteric lymph nodes and presented to B cells. In addition, some bacteria are taken up by specialized antigen-capturing M cells, enter the Peyer patches, and become resident within the tissues. Although most of these invading bacteria are killed by macrophages, some are also presented to B cells. The B cells produce IgA, which may bind to bacteria, modify the composition of the microbiota, and block further mucosal penetration.

Regulatory T Cells

Intestinal helper T (Th) cell precursors can differentiate into either Treg or Th17 cells on receiving signals from the microbiota.[36] In effect, the microbiota collectively programs the T-cell system to optimize its function and so maximize its survival (bear in mind that the host's survival is also of importance to the microbiota).

Intestinal Treg cells are a subset of CD4$^+$ helper cells required to maintain the body's commensal relationship with its microbiota. They produce the suppressive cytokine, IL-10. Treg production occurs in response to signals from both the microbiota and enterocytes. Under stable conditions, the production of Treg cells is favored, whereas that of Th17 cells is suppressed and minimal inflammation occurs within the intestinal wall. In the absence of Treg cells, uncontrolled effector T cells will respond to microbial antigens and trigger inflammation. Mucosal inflammation is therefore actively suppressed by the production of large numbers of IL-10–producing Tregs. IL-10-deficient mice develop chronic unremitting colitis driven by IL-23 and the Th17 pathway.

However, it is also clear that this tolerance can only go so far. Should a potential pathogen seek to invade the body from the intestine, then the immune system must be prepared to act aggressively to prevent this. This is mediated by proinflammatory Th17 cells.

T Helper 17 Cells

Th17 cells are a subset of CD4$^+$ helper cells that promote inflammation. Under the influence of IL-23, they produce the proinflammatory cytokines IL-17 and IL-22. Like Treg cells, the development of Th17 cells is regulated by signals from the microbiota and from enterocytes. Th17 cell development is specifically stimulated by the attachment of segmented filamentous bacteria (SFBs) to enterocytes.[37] Enterocytes can sense this tight attachment and stimulate IL-23 production by macrophages, leading to production of IL-17 and IL-22.[30]

SFBs are unique spore-forming, long filamentous, gram-positive anaerobic commensals found in the small intestine of mammals and birds (although they have yet to be reported in dogs and cats).[38] SFBs stimulate the upregulation of host innate defense genes and inflammatory cytokines. They attach very strongly to the enterocytes of the ileum where they can be sampled by dendritic cells (most other commensal bacteria remain within the mucous layers). SFBs induce the development of germinal centers in Peyer's patches and other intestinal lymphoid organs, and increase production of IgA and Th17 cells.[39]

DYSBIOSIS

If the intestinal microbiota becomes unstable or imbalanced, dysbiosis occurs. It is possible to target specific pathogenic bacterial groups in real time, determine a dysbiosis index using qPCR, and then determine levels of functional microbial metabolites, including bile acids and SCFAs. The Dysbiosis Index developed by the Texas A&M College of Veterinary Medicine Gastrointestinal Laboratory is a rapid PCR-based assay that can be used to quantify 8 different bacterial groups commonly present in the gastrointestinal tract of dogs and cats and express them as a single value that can help indicate the level of dysbiosis. It can also predict normal or abnormal conversion of fecal bile acids, which are affected by alterations in the gastrointestinal microbiota. Dogs show an increase in the Dysbiosis Index in instances of chronic enteropathy, exocrine pancreatic insufficiency, or antibiotic-induced dysbiosis.[3] In many cases, it is not always clear whether this dysbiosis is the cause or the effect of the disease.

The loss of commensal bacterial microbiota has been linked to metabolic changes.[40] Dysbiosis is a cause of equine laminitis[41,42] and bovine ruminal acidosis,[37] and has been implicated in the development of diseases such as canine chronic enteropathy and inflammatory bowel diseases. Antibiotic treatment is an important cause of dysbiosis because it can radically alter the composition of the intestinal microbiota and increase the risk of developing infections with organisms such as *Clostridium difficile* or overgrowth with other unwanted pathogens. Antibiotics can also alter the composition of the microbiota, resulting in an increased risk of obesity (obese individuals have more Firmicutes and fewer *Bacteroides* than lean ones). Perhaps the most significant dysbiosis is that which leads to the development of allergies.[43]

The Hygiene Hypothesis

The prevalence of allergic disease has increased significantly in Western societies over the past 50 years. Although most obvious in humans, this has also affected their pets. It is likely that this increase is, at least partially, a result of changes in their microbiota.[44–49] The hygiene hypothesis suggests that alterations in Western diets, environmental cleanliness, an urban lifestyle, and overuse of antibiotics together cause long-term changes in the intestinal microbiota. Given the close association between pets and humans, it is unsurprising that the microbiota of pets has come to resemble that of humans. Dysbiosis in humans may well be reflected in their pets. Because the intestinal microbiota influences the Th1-Th2 balance, it is suggested that, as a result of this loss of diversity, Th2 responses come to predominate. Thus the composition of the intestinal microbiota exerts a significant influence on allergy development.

The hygiene hypothesis has received support from studies on piglets. Major differences can be found in their gut microbiota depending on the environment in which piglets are raised.[50] These differences also influence the expression of immune system genes. For example, pigs raised in a very clean environment have reduced microbial diversity and express more genes involved in inflammation.

Conversely, outdoor pigs with a diverse microbiota express more genes linked to T-cell function. Similar effects have been observed in rodents. Germ-free mice have high serum IgE levels in early life. These can be greatly reduced by bacterial colonization, suggesting that the microbiota regulate IgE production. If low doses of vancomycin are fed to neonatal mice, the diversity of their gut microbiota is reduced, their Treg numbers are reduced, and they suffer from increased severity of allergic lung disease. Adult mice treated with oral antibiotics have increased IgE levels and blood basophil numbers. They too have increased airway inflammation following allergen challenge.

Conversely, an appropriately balanced microbiota generates antiinflammatory molecules such as SCFAs, polysaccharide A, and peptidoglycans. SCFAs, such as formate, acetate, butyrate, and succinate and glycans, are produced in abundance in high-fiber diets.[51] Human populations that consume large amounts of fiber have a lower prevalence of colitis and inflammatory disease. Among the SCFAs, butyrate has potent antiinflammatory properties and inhibits proinflammatory responses by intestinal macrophages. Butyric acid acts on macrophages and prevents epigenetic changes by inhibiting histone deacetylases. Butyrate also increases barrier functions by stimulating enterocytes and increasing transcription of mucin genes, goblet cell differentiation, and mucous production. It can also stimulate some bovine neutrophil functions. Therefore, a balanced and healthy microbiota suppresses inflammation by stimulating Treg activity.

Intestinal Diseases

Intestinal dysbiosis is often associated with disease development.[3] Chronic enteropathies are a diverse group of diseases that result from a combination of genetic, microbial, nutritional, allergic, and environmental factors. Some resemble inflammatory bowel diseases in humans (Crohn's disease and ulcerative colitis) but most probably have a different pathogenesis.[52] Some result from dysbiosis in the intestinal microbiota. As pointed out, commensal bacteria within the intestine suppress inflammation by generating IL-10–secreting Treg cells. If these control mechanisms fail and the animal responds aggressively to its commensals by increasing Th17 responses, severe inflammation may result.

Canine chronic enteropathies are characterized by persistent or recurrent gastrointestinal inflammation.[52] These usually present with a history of chronic vomiting, diarrhea, or weight loss. There is a breed predisposition in Weimaraners, Rottweilers, German shepherds, border collies, and boxers. The most common form of enteropathy is a lymphocytic-plasmacytic enteritis. Affected dogs show an increase in Proteobacteria, especially E coli or Pseudomonas, and a decrease in Firmicutes and Bacteroidetes. Other changes, such as increased bacterial adherence to the mucosa, reduced bacterial diversity, and overgrowth of other bacteria, may all contribute to the inflammation.[53,54]

Many cases are associated with an increase in T cell and IgA+ plasma cells in the small intestine.[55] Some dogs with chronic enteropathy have reduced IgA levels in feces, duodenum, and blood.

The affected small intestine shows increased messenger RNA for IL-12, IFN-γ, tumor necrosis factor (TNF)-α, and transforming growth factor (TGF)-β. In dogs, cases have been associated with altered expression or dysregulation of TLR-2, TLR-4, and TLR-5. Polymorphisms in TLR-4 and TLR-5 have also been associated with disease susceptibility. Thus it has been suggested that excessive TLR activation might increase IL-1β levels. If this is accompanied by decreased production of its IL-1 receptor antagonist (IL-1RA) then acute inflammation may result. The IL-1RA to IL-1 ratio in affected dogs is negatively correlated with disease severity. There is no evidence for changes in Th17 cell activity in these diseases in dogs. Likewise, there is no evidence of a Th1-Th2 imbalance in either dogs or cats.

In about 50% of canine cases, feeding a hypoallergenic or a novel antigen diet may result in rapid clinical improvement within a few days and suggests that some forms of enteropathy result from food hypersensitivities. Other forms may result from enteric infections and may respond well to antibiotic therapy. Drugs commonly used include oxytetracycline, metronidazole, and tylosin. These responsive dogs include young large-breed animals and German shepherds. The effects of antibiotic therapy may, however, be short-lived.

Some cases are immunologically mediated and dogs may respond well to glucocorticoids, such as prednisolone, and the immunosuppressive drugs, such as cyclosporine or azathioprine. Unfortunately, the results of many clinical trials have been mixed and confusing, so long-term control remains difficult.

Histiocytic ulcerative colitis in boxers is a severe form of inflammatory bowel disease. The lesions are characterized by the presence of large macrophages that stain intensely with periodic acid–Schiff stain. It has been suggested that this colitis is triggered by an unidentified infectious agent because it somewhat resembles Johne's disease. The lesions also show accumulations of plasma cells, macrophages, and granulocytes.

Immunoproliferative enteropathy of Basenjis is an inherited autosomal disease that presents as gastric mucosal hypertrophy with lymphoid cell infiltration and ulceration. The whole small intestine may show villous blunting, crypt elongation, and infiltration of the mucosa with lymphocytes, plasma cells, and some neutrophils. Dogs show a polyclonal increase in serum IgA. The disease may be controlled by high doses of corticosteroids.

Protein-losing enteropathy of soft-coated Wheaten terriers is also an inherited disease. Histologic examination of dogs with this condition shows an inflammatory bowel disease. The cellular infiltrates are mainly lymphocytes and plasma cells, but neutrophils and eosinophils are often present. This disease may result from food hypersensitivity, possibly to wheat gluten.

Gluten-sensitive enteropathy of Irish setters is an autosomal recessive small intestinal disease also caused by exposure to wheat gluten. As with the diseases described previously, affected small intestine is infiltrated with lymphocytes and other inflammatory cells. The mucosa shows increased numbers of CD4$^+$ cells and decreased CD8$^+$ T-cell numbers. Affected dogs may also have elevated serum IgA levels.

Lymphocytic-plasmacytic enteritis has also been described in cats, horses, and a cow.

Respiratory Disease

The airway microbiota plays a role in resistance to respiratory infections and development of asthma and chronic obstructive pulmonary disease. Thus, in the absence of a microbiota, the airways are prone to mount exaggerated Th2 responses. The presence of the microbiota induces Treg activity. This probably explains the protective effects of inhaled microbial antigens on the development of allergies in children. Dietary fiber also has a protective effect on allergic airway inflammation in mice as a result of increased levels of SCFAs. The intestinal microbiota also regulates pulmonary adaptive responses.[18] Thus SFBs in the intestine regulate pulmonary immunity to bacteria and fungi. Conversely, influenza infection in the lungs generates type I interferons that, in turn, induce intestinal dysbiosis, such as depletion of obligate anaerobic bacteria and an increase in Proteobacteria.[19]

Atopic Dermatitis

The intestinal and skin surfaces have much in common and interact extensively. The intestinal microbiota with its huge numbers of metabolites may well induce cutaneous changes. The most significant mechanism is through alterations in the Th17-Treg balance, whereas other effects may be mediated by retinoic acid or vitamin A and vitamin D and neuroendocrine interactions.[56,57]

AD is therefore associated with dysbiosis both in the skin and the intestine.[17,58] The skin microbiome seems to influence skin barrier function.[59] Staphylococcal colonization correlates with changes in skin barrier function; when the infection was treated and normal microbial diversity restored, normal function was also restored.[59]

Intestinal dysbiosis also affects the development of AD and manipulation of the intestinal microbiota may assist in the treatment of this disease. Obviously, food allergies may be directly involved in the pathogenesis of atopic skin disease. However, changes in the gut microbiota also influence the level of allergic and inflammatory responses through changes in the Th17-Treg balance. The intestinal microbiota differs from normal in humans with AD,[60] and systemic antibiotic treatment increases the risk of AD in humans.[61] Early exposure to some probiotics can have both short-term and long-term effects on dogs with AD.[62–64]

Autoimmunity

Because the gut microbiota influences the development of immunologic tolerance, dysbiosis may also affect the development of autoimmune disease.[65,66] For example, nonobese diabetic (NOD) mice develop spontaneous insulin-dependent diabetes mellitus associated with infiltration of the pancreatic islets by lymphocytes. Their disease resembles human type 1 diabetes mellitus. Its development is influenced by their microbiota. Thus conventional NOD mice that lack MyD88 protein (MyD88 is an adaptor molecule for the TLRs) do not develop diabetes, whereas totally germ-free MyD88⁻ NOD mice do. If commensal bacteria are given to these germ-free mice, their diabetes is less severe. Somehow, the interaction of the intestinal microbiota with the immune system influences the predisposition of these mice to develop diabetes.

Alterations in the intestinal microbiota also influence autoimmune diseases such as rheumatoid arthritis, ankylosing spondylitis, insulin-dependent diabetes mellitus, and experimental autoimmune encephalitis.[67] In some mouse arthritis models, changes in the gut microbiota due to antibiotic treatment can exacerbate the disease. Antinuclear antibody production in mice is influenced by the microbiota, especially by increased colonization with SFB.

SUMMARY

The presence of huge numbers of microbes on body surfaces provides a rich source of signals to the immune system. Given that animals have evolved in the presence of the microbiota, it is unsurprising that the immune system has come to depend on these signals and that changes in the microbiota will provoke changes in these signals that result in alterations in immune function. The mutualistic partnership has evolved to conserve microbial signaling and immune response pathways to ensure an animal's survival in a world dominated by microbes.[51,68] Given the close interactions between the intestine, the respiratory tract, and the skin, it is to be expected that dysbiosis may affect all 3 surfaces or systems. The growing body of data on this subject will likely provide a fruitful source of ideas regarding the prevention and treatment of a multitude of immunologic diseases in domestic mammals.

REFERENCES

1. Arpaia N, Rudensky AY. Microbial metabolites control gut inflammatory responses. Proc Natl Acad Sci U S A 2014;111(6):2058–9.
2. Hand TW. The role of the microbiota in shaping infectious immunity. Trends Immunol 2016;37(10):647–58.
3. Suchodolski JS. Diagnosis and interpretation of intestinal dysbiosis in dogs and cats. Vet J 2016;215:30–7.
4. Hooda S, Minamoto Y, Suchodolski JS, et al. Current state of knowledge: the canine gastrointestinal microbiome. Anim Health Res Rev 2012;13(1):78–88.
5. Costa MC, Silva G, Ramos RV, et al. Characterization and comparison of the bacterial microbiota in different gastrointestinal tract compartments in horses. Vet J 2015;205(1):74–80.
6. Suchodolski JS. Intestinal microbiota of dogs and cats: a bigger world than we thought. Vet Clin North Am Small Anim Pract 2011;41(2):261–72.
7. Garcia-Mazcorro JF, Castillo-Carranza SA, Guard B, et al. Comprehensive molecular characterization of bacterial communities in feces of pet birds using 16S marker sequencing. Microb Ecol 2017;73(1):224–35.
8. Handl S, Dowd SE, Garcia-Mazcorro JF, et al. Massive parallel 16S rRNA gene pyrosequencing reveals highly diverse fecal bacterial and fungal communities in healthy dogs and cats. FEMS Microbiol Ecol 2011;76(2):301–10.
9. Tamburini S, Shen N, Wu HC, et al. The microbiome in early life: implications for health outcomes. Nat Med 2016;22(7):713–22.
10. Gensollen T, Iyer SS, Kasper DL, et al. How colonization by microbiota in early life shapes the immune system. Science 2016;352(6285):539–44.
11. Brown RL, Clarke TB. The regulation of host defences to infection by the microbiota. Immunology 2016;150(1):1–6.
12. Kong HH. Skin microbiome: genomics-based insights into the diversity and role of skin microbes. Trends Mol Med 2011;17(6):320–8.
13. Rodrigues Hoffmann A, Patterson AP, Diesel A, et al. The skin microbiome in healthy and allergic dogs. PLoS One 2014;9(1):e83197.
14. Verwoerd DJ. Ostrich diseases. Rev Sci Tech 2000;19(2):638–61.
15. Older CE, Diesel A, Patterson AP, et al. The feline skin microbiota: the bacteria inhabiting the skin of healthy and allergic cats. PLoS One 2017;12(6):e0178555.
16. Gallo RL, Hooper LV. Epithelial antimicrobial defence of the skin and intestine. Nat Rev Immunol 2012;12(7):503–16.
17. Kennedy EA, Connolly J, Hourihane JO, et al. Skin microbiome before development of atopic dermatitis: early colonization with commensal staphylococci at 2 months is associated with a lower risk of atopic dermatitis at 1 year. J Allergy Clin Immunol 2017;139(1):166–72.
18. O'Dwyer DN, Dickson RP, Moore BB. The lung microbiome, immunity, and the pathogenesis of chronic lung disease. J Immunol 2016;196(12):4839–47.
19. Tamburini S, Clemente JC. Gut microbiota: neonatal gut microbiota induces lung immunity against pneumonia. Nat Rev Gastroenterol Hepatol 2017;14(5):263–4.
20. Deng P, Swanson KS. Gut microbiota of humans, dogs and cats: current knowledge and future opportunities and challenges. Br J Nutr 2015;113(Suppl):S6–17.
21. Kamada N, Chen GY, Inohara N, et al. Control of pathogens and pathobionts by the gut microbiota. Nat Immunol 2013;14(7):685–90.
22. Kamada N, Seo SU, Chen GY, et al. Role of the gut microbiota in immunity and inflammatory disease. Nat Rev Immunol 2013;13(5):321–35.

23. Geva-Zatorsky N, Sefik E, Kua L, et al. Mining the human gut microbiota for immunomodulatory organisms. Cell 2017;168(5):928–43.e11.

24. Kamada N, Nunez G. Role of the gut microbiota in the development and function of lymphoid cells. J Immunol 2013;190(4):1389–95.

25. Butler JE, Santiago-Mateo K, Wertz N, et al. Antibody repertoire development in fetal and neonatal piglets. XXIV. Hypothesis: the ileal Peyer patches (IPP) are the major source of primary, undiversified IgA antibodies in newborn piglets. Developmental Comp Immunol 2016;65:340–51.

26. Butler JE, Sinkora M. The enigma of the lower gut-associated lymphoid tissue (GALT). J Leukoc Biol 2013;94(2):259–70.

27. Rhee KJ, Sethupathi P, Driks A, et al. Role of commensal bacteria in development of gut-associated lymphoid tissues and preimmune antibody repertoire. J Immunol 2004;172(2):1118–24.

28. Tomkovich S, Jobin C. Microbiota and host immune responses: a love-hate relationship. Immunology 2016;147(1):1–10.

29. McDermott AJ, Huffnagle GB. The microbiome and regulation of mucosal immunity. Immunology 2014;142(1):24–31.

30. Gaboriau-Routhiau V, Rakotobe S, Lecuyer E, et al. The key role of segmented filamentous bacteria in the coordinated maturation of gut helper T cell responses. Immunity 2009;31(4):677–89.

31. Peterson LW, Artis D. Intestinal epithelial cells: regulators of barrier function and immune homeostasis. Nat Rev Immunol 2014;14(3):141–53.

32. Eberl G, Colonna M, Di Santo JP, et al. Innate lymphoid cells. Innate lymphoid cells: a new paradigm in immunology. Science 2015;348(6237):aaa6566.

33. Hepworth MR, Fung TC, Masur SH, et al. Immune tolerance. Group 3 innate lymphoid cells mediate intestinal selection of commensal bacteria-specific CD4(+) T cells. Science 2015;348(6238):1031–5.

34. Hepworth MR, Monticelli LA, Fung TC, et al. Innate lymphoid cells regulate CD4+ T-cell responses to intestinal commensal bacteria. Nature 2013;498(7452):113–7.

35. Gury-BenAri M, Thaiss CA, Serafini N, et al. The spectrum and regulatory landscape of intestinal innate lymphoid cells are shaped by the microbiome. Cell 2016;166(5):1231–46.e13.

36. Ohnmacht C, Park JH, Cording S, et al. Mucosal immunology. The microbiota regulates type 2 immunity through RORgammat(+) T cells. Science 2015;349(6251): 989–93.

37. Schnupf P, Gaboriau-Routhiau V, Gros M, et al. Growth and host interaction of mouse segmented filamentous bacteria in vitro. Nature 2015;520(7545):99–103.

38. Lecuyer E, Rakotobe S, Lengline-Garnier H, et al. Segmented filamentous bacterium uses secondary and tertiary lymphoid tissues to induce gut IgA and specific T helper 17 cell responses. Immunity 2014;40(4):608–20.

39. Ivanov II, Honda K. Intestinal commensal microbes as immune modulators. Cell Host Microbe 2012;12(4):496–508.

40. Sansonetti PJ, Di Santo JP. Debugging how bacteria manipulate the immune response. Immunity 2007;26(2):149–61.

41. Katz LM, Bailey SR. A review of recent advances and current hypotheses on the pathogenesis of acute laminitis. Equine Vet J 2012;44(6):752–61.

42. Plaizier JC, Li S, Danscher AM, et al. Changes in microbiota in rumen digesta and feces due to a grain-based subacute ruminal acidosis (SARA) challenge. Microb Ecol 2017;74(2):485–95.

43. Becattini S, Taur Y, Pamer EG. Antibiotic-induced changes in the intestinal microbiota and disease. Trends Mol Med 2016;22(6):458–78.

44. Belkaid Y, Hand TW. Role of the microbiota in immunity and inflammation. Cell 2014;157(1):121–41.
45. Flohr C, Yeo L. Atopic dermatitis and the hygiene hypothesis revisited. Curr Probl Dermatol 2011;41:1–34.
46. Kantor R, Silverberg JI. Environmental risk factors and their role in the management of atopic dermatitis. Expert Rev Clin Immunol 2017;13(1):15–26.
47. Bloomfield SF, Rook GA, Scott EA, et al. Time to abandon the hygiene hypothesis: new perspectives on allergic disease, the human microbiome, infectious disease prevention and the role of targeted hygiene. Perspect Public Health 2016;136(4): 213–24.
48. Maizels RM. Parasitic helminth infections and the control of human allergic and autoimmune disorders. Clin Microbiol Infect 2016;22(6):481–6.
49. Thomas CL, Fernandez-Penas P. The microbiome and atopic eczema: more than skin deep. Australas J Dermatol 2017;58(1):18–24.
50. Mulder IE, Schmidt B, Stokes CR, et al. Environmentally-acquired bacteria influence microbial diversity and natural innate immune responses at gut surfaces. BMC Biol 2009;7:79.
51. Rooks MG, Garrett WS. Gut microbiota, metabolites and host immunity. Nat Rev Immunol 2016;16(6):341–52.
52. Dandrieux JR. Inflammatory bowel disease versus chronic enteropathy in dogs: are they one and the same? J Small Anim Pract 2016;57(11):589–99.
53. Xenoulis PG, Palculict B, Allenspach K, et al. Molecular-phylogenetic characterization of microbial communities imbalances in the small intestine of dogs with inflammatory bowel disease. FEMS Microbiol Ecol 2008;66(3):579–89.
54. Suchodolski JS, Xenoulis PG, Paddock CG, et al. Molecular analysis of the bacterial microbiota in duodenal biopsies from dogs with idiopathic inflammatory bowel disease. Vet Microbiol 2010;142(3–4):394–400.
55. Ridyard AE, Nuttall TJ, Else RW, et al. Evaluation of Th1, Th2 and immunosuppressive cytokine mRNA expression within the colonic mucosa of dogs with idiopathic lymphocytic-plasmacytic colitis. Vet Immunol Immunopathol 2002;86(3–4): 205–14.
56. O'Neill CA, Monteleone G, McLaughlin JT, et al. The gut-skin axis in health and disease: a paradigm with therapeutic implications. Bioessays 2016;38(11): 1167–76.
57. Plunkett CH, Nagler CR. The influence of the microbiome on allergic sensitization to food. J Immunol 2017;198(2):581–9.
58. Kobayashi T, Glatz M, Horiuchi K, et al. Dysbiosis and staphylococcus aureus colonization drives inflammation in atopic dermatitis. Immunity 2015;42(4): 756–66.
59. Bradley CW, Morris DO, Rankin SC, et al. Longitudinal evaluation of the skin microbiome and association with microenvironment and treatment in canine atopic dermatitis. J Invest Dermatol 2016;136(6):1182–90.
60. Watanabe S, Narisawa Y, Arase S, et al. Differences in fecal microflora between patients with atopic dermatitis and healthy control subjects. J Allergy Clin Immunol 2003;111(3):587–91.
61. Tsakok T, McKeever TM, Yeo L, et al. Does early life exposure to antibiotics increase the risk of eczema? A systematic review. Br J Dermatol 2013;169(5): 983–91.
62. Marsella R. Evaluation of Lactobacillus rhamnosus strain GG for the prevention of atopic dermatitis in dogs. Am J Vet Res 2009;70(6):735–40.

63. Marsella R, Santoro D, Ahrens K. Early exposure to probiotics in a canine model of atopic dermatitis has long-term clinical and immunological effects. Vet Immunol Immunopathol 2012;146(2):185–9.

64. Grzeskowiak L, Endo A, Beasley S, et al. Microbiota and probiotics in canine and feline welfare. Anaerobe 2015;34:14–23.

65. Yurkovetskiy LA, Pickard JM, Chervonsky AV. Microbiota and autoimmunity: exploring new avenues. Cell Host Microbe 2015;17(5):548–52.

66. Van Praet JT, Donovan E, Vanassche I, et al. Commensal microbiota influence systemic autoimmune responses. EMBO J 2015;34(4):466–74.

67. Wu HJ, Ivanov II, Darce J, et al. Gut-residing segmented filamentous bacteria drive autoimmune arthritis via T helper 17 cells. Immunity 2010;32(6):815–27.

68. Blacher E, Levy M, Tatirovsky E, et al. Microbiome-modulated metabolites at the interface of host immunity. J Immunol 2017;198(2):572–80.

Current and Newly Emerging Autoimmune Diseases

Laurel J. Gershwin, DVM, PhD

KEYWORDS

- Autoimmunity • Self-tolerance • Autoantibodies • Self-reactive T cells

KEY POINTS

- There are many autoimmune diseases that are recognized in domestic animals.
- The descriptions of diseases provide examples of the magnitude of immune targets and the variable nature of autoimmune diseases.
- Autoimmune diseases recognized in dogs, cats, and horses can affect single or multiple body systems including skin, blood (anemia), endocrine, ocular, and neuromuscular.

INTRODUCTION
Autoimmunity: Horror Autotoxicus

The immune system is designed to permit discrimination between cells and tissues defined as self and infectious agents, so that the strong and effective mechanisms for causing destruction of potential pathogens or other elements foreign to the host are properly targeted. When these defense mechanisms are instead directed against the host, autoimmune disease results. This concept of horror autotoxicus was coined by Dr Paul Ehrlich in the early 1900s. Shortly thereafter the first autoimmune diseases were described.[1] Thus, autoimmune diseases are caused by the stimulation of an immune response that reacts with self. There are a variety of ways that this can occur, some well recognized and others not yet determined.[2,3] It is known that inheritance of certain genes can influence susceptibility to autoimmune diseases and that environmental factors can interact with the immune system of the host to precipitate autoimmunity. The increased incidence of some autoimmune diseases in certain dog or cat breeds shows that inbreeding can increase the frequency of genotypes that are associated with those autoimmune conditions. Many well-defined human autoimmune diseases, such as immune-mediated anemia and autoimmune thyroiditis (Hashimoto's thyroiditis), have been recognized in dogs for many years, whereas other diseases are currently under investigation as potentially having an autoimmune cause.

Disclosure: The authors have nothing to disclose.
Department of Pathology, Microbiology and Immunology, School of Veterinary Medicine, University of California, Davis, Vet Med 3A, Davis, CA 95616, USA
E-mail address: ljgershwin@ucdavis.edu

Vet Clin Small Anim 48 (2018) 323–338
https://doi.org/10.1016/j.cvsm.2017.10.010
0195-5616/18/© 2017 Elsevier Inc. All rights reserved.

Development of Self-Tolerance

Development of self-tolerance involves both central and peripheral mechanisms; these may eliminate or suppress self-reactive lymphocytes, thereby preventing immune recognition of self. Central tolerance occurs during fetal life. The thymus is an important organ of the immune system, and during fetal life it is responsible for removing T lymphocytes that are capable of binding with high affinity to self-peptides. After entering the thymus from the bone marrow, T lymphocytes acquire T-cell receptors in the thymic cortex. Once these cells enter the thymic medulla their receptors are tested for reactivity with self-peptides and are negatively selected if they show a high affinity for self-antigens. In this process T cells whose receptors bind tightly to the self are stimulated to undergo apoptosis and they die. The remaining T cells with a moderate affinity for self are preserved.[2] Moderate affinity is required because self-recognition in the context of a normal immune response is required.[2]

Besides the major histocompatibility determinants that are definitive for cells from an individual (and therefore determine what is self), there are organ-specific molecules that the immune system must not recognize as foreign. To tolerize the T cells to these organ-specific determinants/antigens the thymic epithelium expresses these multiple determinants that are present on organs of the body. A gene called the Aire gene is referred to as an autoimmune regulator. It is a transcription factor responsible for the expression of these self-proteins on the medullary epithelial cells. This ability to express multiple antigens in the thymus during fetal development allows the remaining T-cell population to be screened for nonreactivity with self-determinants on various tissues and cells in the body. In some human patients a genetic defect in the Aire gene has been described and linked with the disease called autoimmune polyendocrine syndrome type 1.[2]

Despite the expression of self-determinants in the thymus and the selection of T lymphocytes that occurs there, the depletion of self-reactive T lymphocytes is not complete. There are, however, other mechanisms that maintain tolerance, such as T-regulatory cells. The T-regulatory cells have the cell surface markers CD4+, CD25+, and the transcription factor fox P3. These cells operate by production of cytokines that can suppress the immune response.[2]

B lymphocytes develop in the bone marrow of mammals and there they acquire receptors that bind to foreign antigens. Self-tolerance in the B-cell population occurs through several mechanisms, including clonal deletion, anergy, and receptor editing.[2] But B cells require T-cell help for initiation of antibody production (with the exception of T-independent antigens, which can stimulate immunoglobulin [Ig] M only). Thus, in the absence of self-reactive T cells, a potentially self-reactive B cell is held in check and does not proliferate and produce self-reactive antibodies. On occasion, B cells can produce autoantibodies after activation of T cells that recognize an epitope cross-reactive with the host's tissues and are thereby able to act as helpers for B cells with receptors for epitopes on that antigen.[2]

Autoimmune Diseases

Autoimmune diseases can be classified by body systems that are affected. Some conditions influence multiple body systems, whereas others affect only one organ. There are several lupuslike syndromes described in human patients as well as the well-defined disease systemic lupus erythematosus (SLE), a multisystemic autoimmune disease. There are examples of both multisystem and organ-specific autoimmune diseases in dogs, cats, and horses. The more specific autoimmune diseases that affect a single type of cell, such as immune-mediated anemia and immune-mediated thrombocytopenia, are among the more common autoimmune diseases seen in dogs. Other autoimmune diseases affect a single organ but may have multiple antigens that are targeted within that organ. Hashimoto's thyroiditis is one example.[3]

It is well established that there is a genetic predisposition for some autoimmune diseases. In human patients the linkage is usually through a major histocompatibility gene. In dogs it is common for certain breeds to have a higher or lower incidence of certain autoimmune diseases and, when dog leukocyte antigens (DLA) are evaluated, it is usually found that certain alleles are more prevalent in affected than in unaffected animals. A more detailed description of these associations is presented with each disease.

Treatment of autoimmune diseases generally involves overall suppression of the immune system. This generalization is true for immune-mediated anemia, thrombocytopenia, and SLE. For some autoimmune diseases (hypothyroidism, hypoadrenocorticism, and diabetes mellitus) lifetime supplementation of the hormone rendered deficient by autoimmune destruction of cells that produce the hormone must be used. Individual treatment options are discussed for specific diseases.

Common Autoimmune Diseases of Dogs

Immune-mediated (hemolytic) anemia
Description and pathogenesis The most common autoimmune disease of dogs is immune-mediated hemolytic anemia (IMHA). This disease is associated with significant morbidity and mortality. Autoantibodies that bind to erythrocytes and cause anemia by a type 2 hypersensitivity mechanism are produced (**Fig. 1**). The isotype of the antibodies influences the type of clinical presentation. For example, if IgM antibodies

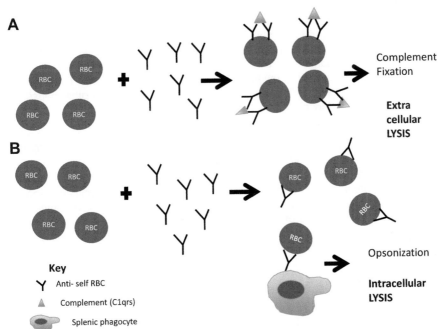

Fig. 1. (*A*) Autoantibodies bind to erythrocytes with Fab segments, fix complement, and initiate the lysis of the target cell (the erythrocyte). Two IgG molecules are required to bind the C1q complement protein to initiate the cascade, but only a single IgM molecule is required for initiation. (*B*) Erythrocytes opsonized with IgG antibodies are removed from circulation and destroyed by fixed macrophages in the spleen. RBC, red blood cell.

are made, the fixation of complement and lysis of the red blood cells is the major outcome, resulting in hemolysis. However, if IgG is produced the outcome may be nonhemolytic with erythrocyte destruction occurring by opsonization and phagocytosis, decreasing the hematocrit without lysis. Splenomegaly is commonly associated with immune-mediated anemia. Breed predisposition for IMHA includes cocker spaniels, Irish setters, Old English sheepdogs, Samoyeds, miniature dachshunds, Scottish terriers, and vizslas.[3]

Primary idiopathic immune-mediated anemia is usually not traced to a single causal factor, although genetic predisposition and potential environmental factors are often implicated. In contrast, secondary immune-mediated anemia is frequently traceable to an underlying cause, most commonly treatment with a drug. Some drugs (including antibiotics) can be metabolized into small molecules that act as haptens and bind to the patient's erythrocytes to elicit antibody production. A good history from the owner, including recent drugs the dog may have been taking, is important information to assist in determining whether the anemia is primary or secondary. If a drug is identified as a causal factor, discontinuation of the drug will ultimately stop erythrocyte lysis (once the affected cells are gone).

Diagnosis Diagnosis of immune-mediated (hemolytic) anemia begins with examination of the patient. The dog is lethargic and shows either very pale or yellow (icteric) mucous membranes. A normal body temperature is common, but the respiratory rate is generally increased and a tachycardia is present. On occasion patients present after acute collapse. On examination of the blood the hematocrit is very low. There is often notable spherocytosis of the erythrocytes as well as reticulocytosis. If icterus is present, the plasma bilirubin level will be increased. Hemoglobinuria may be visualized if active hemolysis has occurred. Autoagglutination of erythrocytes is also a common observation.

Laboratory diagnosis of IMHA should include the performance of a Coombs test, which reveals the presence of antierythrocyte antibodies bound to the red blood cells (direct Coombs) and sometimes also circulating antierythrocyte antibodies (indirect Coombs). This test is used to show the presence of the autoantibodies. These results are critical for the differentiation of immune-mediated anemia from other causes of anemia, such as blood loss or bone marrow suppression.[4]

Treatment Mortality from IMHA is high, often close to 50%. Therapy involves both modulation of the immune response and adjunctive therapy to treat the presenting signs. A blood transfusion may be required to save the patient from a terminal outcome before immunosuppressive drugs can be given. The initial drug of choice is often a glucocorticoid (such as prednisone, prednisolone, or dexamethasone). The antiinflammatory effects of glucocorticoids reduce the destruction of opsonized erythrocytes by macrophages. Higher doses of prednisone are required for immunosuppression (2–4 mg/kg/d). Other immunosuppressive drugs may be used in combination with prednisone or alone. These drugs include cyclophosphamide and azathioprine.[5]

Autoimmune Endocrine Diseases

Several endocrine organs are targeted by autoimmune disease: the endocrine pancreas (islet cells), the thyroid gland, and the adrenal gland. Diabetes mellitus, thyroiditis, and hypoadrenocorticism (Addison disease) are caused by immune attack on cells that are essential for production of hormones. Often the disease process is not recognized until sufficient cell death has occurred to create a deficit of the hormone produced by that organ. For this reason, therapy for these diseases is directed less at immunosuppression and more at hormone replacement therapy.

Autoimmune thyroiditis

Description and pathogenesis The most common autoimmune endocrine disease in dogs is thyroiditis with consequent hypothyroidism. It is also the most common auto-immune disease in humans; Hashimoto thyroiditis and autoimmune thyroiditis in dogs have many similarities. A loss of tolerance to thyroid proteins causes destruction of thyroid follicular cells and specific antibody responses to thyroglobulin (the prohormone for production of T3 and T4). A second target protein is thyroid peroxidase, which is required for thyroid hormone synthesis. The thyroid-stimulating hormone receptor (TSHR) is the third major antigenic target in human thyroiditis.[6]

Unlike many autoimmune diseases that can have life-threatening consequences, patients with this disorder can lead normal lives with daily supplementation of thyroxin.

The clinical presentation of a dog with hypothyroidism generally involves lethargy, dullness, weight gain, and sometimes dermatologic changes, such as hair loss and otitis. A moderate anemia may also be present. Approximately 50% of hypothyroid dogs have an immune-mediated cause. Laboratory testing for T4, TSH, and antibodies specific for thyroglobulin should be performed. Low T4 and high TSH levels indicate hypothyroidism; the presence of antibodies against thyroglobulin clinches the diagnosis of an autoimmune causation.

The pathogenesis of immune-mediated thyroiditis is thought to involve primarily a T cell–mediated attack on the medullary cells of the thyroid gland with resultant death of those cells that produce thyroxin. Biopsy of an affected thyroid or histopathologic analysis of samples taken at necropsy show infiltration of the gland with lymphocytes [3 and 4]. The presence of the antibodies against thyroglobulin may play a secondary role and/or be simply an indication of the loss of tolerance for both T and B cells.

Diagnosis When the clinical signs indicate hypothyroidism (lethargy, weight gain, and seborrhea and/or hair loss), appropriate laboratory analysis should be performed. This analysis includes a thyroid panel consisting of levels of TSH, T4, and thyroglobulin antibody (TG-A). A high TSH level and low T4 level are consistent with the immune-mediated thyroiditis. The presence of antibodies against thyroglobulin and T4 may also be detected.

Treatment Treatment of dogs with hypothyroidism requires daily supplementation with thyroid hormone. It is important to check T4 levels after the patient has been on therapy for several weeks because excess thyroid hormone can lead to thyrotoxicosis.

Diabetes mellitus

Description and pathogenesis Diabetes mellitus is common in both dogs and cats. It resembles diabetes in humans and is classified similarly. In dogs, diabetes mellitus is most often type 1 (autoimmune), and is characterized by the presence of persistent hyperglycemia, polydipsia, polyuria, glucosuria, polyphagia, and weight loss. There is a definite genetic predisposition, which is manifested most in purebred dog breeds. Breeds with a high odds ratio for development of diabetes mellitus include Samoyed (3.36), giant schnauzer (4.78), fox terrier (3.02), and miniature poodle (1.79). Other breeds are less likely to develop diabetes; these include the boxer, with an odds ratio of 0.07. There are numerous other factors that contribute to development of this disease, including concurrent infection, treatment with glucocorticoids, pancreatitis, and obesity.[7]

In cats, diabetes is more similar to type 2 diabetes (not autoimmune) in humans, with approximately 80% of the cases resembling type 2 diabetes. Type 1 diabetes does occur in cats, but it is rare.

Diagnosis By the time that clinical signs of diabetes are apparent, canine patients are showing glucosuria and hyperglycemia. Circulating antibodies against islet cells, insulin, and several other related antigens are often present. In undiagnosed and thus untreated dogs, ketosis can occur.

Treatment Immune-mediated destruction of the pancreatic beta cells results in permanent loss of the ability to produce insulin. Once diagnosed, diabetic dogs must be on lifelong insulin therapy. There are a variety of insulin preparations available and most veterinarians have their preferred product. Whichever insulin is used, continual daily injections must be provided for the remainder of the dog's life.

Hypoadrenocorticism

Hypoadrenocorticism (Addison disease) is an autoimmune disease that is recognized in both humans and dogs. Affected dogs show a deficiency in production of corticosteroid hormones (cortisol and aldosterone) that are normally produced by the adrenal gland. The clinical signs are often nonspecific (vomiting, diarrhea, anorexia, lethargy, weakness) and may be intermittent. As seen with several other autoimmune diseases, there is a genetic predisposition. The incidence of hypoadrenocorticism is increased in several breeds (eg, Portuguese water dogs, Great Danes, standard poodles, West Highland white terriers, and Nova Scotia duck tolling retrievers).[8]

Diagnosis Cortisol levels are low in affected dogs, but the diagnosis is generally made with the adrenocorticotropic hormone (ACTH) stimulation test, which shows an inability to secrete cortisol. In affected patients, the before and after ACTH stimulation cortisol levels are less than 2 µg/dL. Electrolyte imbalance is generally present with a sodium/potassium ratio of less than 27:1.[8] Antibodies to adrenal-associated antigens are found in human patients with Addison disease. In dogs, studies have shown the presence of autoantibodies against P450scc (cytochrome P450 side chain cleavage enzyme).[8] When necropsy samples are available, lymphocytic-plasmacytic inflammation is present in the adrenal cortex.

Treatment Treatment of canine Addison disease involves replacement of the needed hormones: the glucocorticoids and the mineralocorticoids. In an acute episode, the patient may require intravenous fluids to correct electrolyte imbalances and intravenous dexamethasone. For daily treatment, a glucocorticoid such as prednisolone and a mineralocorticoid such as fludrocortisone are given orally.

Polyglandular endocrinopathy type II (schmidt syndrome)

Description and pathogenesis The presence of autoimmune disease of more than one endocrine gland in a single patient is not common, but it is recognized in humans. There is evidence for the occurrence of this syndrome in dogs. One case report describes a 3-year-old female neutered Doberman pinscher. She was presented for lethargy, episodic collapse, ataxia, and myxedema.[9] In another case, an 8-year-old spayed female boxer presented with progressive symmetric alopecia, lethargy, and intolerance to cold.[10]

Diagnosis The diagnosis of hypothyroidism and hypoadrenocorticism (Addison disease) in the first case was based on clinical signs, inadequate response to thyroid hormone replacement, and the finding of autoantibodies to thyroglobulin and 21-hydroxylase in the serum.[9] In the boxer dog there was a low plasma thyroxine level and non-TSH responsiveness. This boxer dog died and, at necropsy, thyroid atrophy and lymphocytic adrenalitis were observed. Both the zona fasciculate and zona reticularis of the adrenal gland were destroyed. The plasma electrolyte concentrations in this dog did not suggest that mineralocorticoid deficiency was involved.[10]

Treatment Treatment of the polyglandular endocrinopathy involves treating for both the hypothyroidism and the hypoadrenocorticism with appropriate hormone replacement, as indicated elsewhere in this article.

Neuromuscular Autoimmune Disease

Myasthenia gravis

Description and pathogenesis Myasthenia gravis (MG) is an autoimmune disease in which there is a development of autoantibodies against the acetylcholine neuroendplate receptor. In normal animals, muscular contraction is initiated when acetyl choline is released at the neuromuscular synapse and binds to its receptor. In this disease, there is an autoimmune attack on the receptors; antibodies bind and elicit a type II hypersensitivity mechanism, which results in complement-mediated destruction of the receptor (**Fig. 2**). When the released acetyl choline is unable to bind to the receptor it results in a diminished or nonexistent contraction of the muscle caused by impaired neuromuscular transmission.

The clinical appearance of patients with this disease involves neuromuscular weakness, which may develop acutely and result in eventual inability to stand. It is also common for canine patients with MG to regurgitate food and water because of a laxity in the muscle of the esophagus (megaesophagus).[11]

MG occurs in cats but is less common than in dogs. In cats with MG, the development of megaesophagus is less common than in dogs. Also in cats, in approximately 50% of cases in one large study of 235 cats there was an association with a mediastinal mass (usually a thymoma).[12]

As with other autoimmune diseases, there is a genetic predisposition; in dogs, the Newfoundland and the Great Dane have an increased MG incidence.[13] Genotyping studies on Newfoundland dogs with early-onset MG (similar to the disease in humans) have identified 3 DLA class II genes linked to a high risk of MG development. These are DLA-DRB1, DLA-DQA1, and DLA-DQB1. These associations were not shared with any other breeds that have a high incidence of MG.[12] In cats, the odds ratio for development of MG is highest in Somali cats (11.6) and also the Abyssinian breed (4.97).[12]

Diagnosis The diagnosis of MG can be made by performing an edrophonium chloride challenge test. This test involves injecting edrophonium chloride (Tensilon) intravenously. Almost immediately an increase in muscle strength is observed and dogs who were unable to rise can get up and walk. Tensilon inhibits the breakdown of acetylcholine so any small amount that is able to bind the few remaining receptors remains at the neuromuscular junction and stimulates the muscle. There are also in vitro assays such as evaluation of the presence of autoantibodies, either circulating or bound to the receptors on biopsy tissue. These autoantibodies are detectable in both canine and feline patients.[11]

Treatment When the esophagus is affected and megaesophagus has been documented, patients can be helped by the construction of a chair in which the dog sits in a vertical position to eat. Anticholinesterase drugs are the cornerstone of therapy; by preventing the metabolism of acetylcholine, the few receptors remaining are able to continue transmitting a signal. Pyridostigmine bromide is commonly used for this function. Sometimes it is necessary to add an immunosuppressive drug such as a corticosteroid to the treatment regime for prevention of continued receptor destruction.[13] In cats that present with a mediastinal mass/thymoma, surgical resection is often performed.[12]

Meningoencephalomyelitis of Unknown Origin

Description and pathogenesis

Meningoencephalomyelitis (MUO) of unknown origin is common in dogs. It is being recognized as an immune-mediated disease that is similar to experimental autoimmune

Normal Neuromuscular Junction

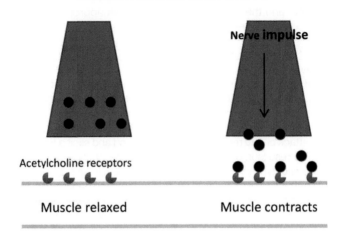

Acetylcholine receptors

Muscle relaxed

Muscle contracts

Myasthenia Gravis

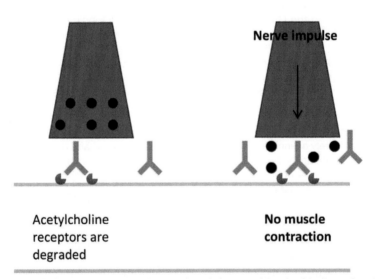

Acetylcholine
receptors are
degraded

**No muscle
contraction**

Fig. 2. Acetyl choline receptors are damaged and destroyed by the binding of antibodies and subsequent complement fixation. Acetylcholine molecules released from the neurons at the neuromuscular synapse are unable to find receptors to bind to before they are rapidly inactivated. Prevention of the metabolism of acetylcholine by stopping cholinesterase activity allows the acetylcholine to stay around long enough to find the few remaining receptors and to bind with resultant muscular contraction.

encephalitis (a condition that is induced experimentally in rodents) and is potentially a good model for multiple sclerosis in human patients. Dogs with MUO may present with signs of central nervous system (CNS) diseases such as seizures or vestibular problems.[14] The literature discusses 3 different diseases, which are often grouped into the category of noninfectious MUO in dogs: granulomatous MUO, necrotizing encephalitis, and meningoencephalitis of unknown origin.[14] The Chihuahua, West Highland white terrier, and Dachshund seem to be over-represented among patients with MUO. However, the pug, Yorkshire terrier, Maltese, Chihuahua, and shih tzu represent 96% of dogs diagnosed with necrotizing encephalitis in a large study on all 3 categories of noninfectious MUO.[14] Genetic risk factors for necrotizing meningoencephalitis have been identified in Maltese dogs on chromosome 4 and chromosome 15 and DLA II loci. Furthermore, fine mapping of these regions showed a potential involvement of ILR7 (interleukin 7 receptor) and FBXW7 (F-box and WD repeat domain containing 7), which are important in immune regulation and have been implicated in multiple sclerosis.[15]

Diagnosis
The clinical signs associated with MUO are related to CNS disease, such as seizures, and brainstem dysfunction including vestibular issues, without evidence of infectious causation. A variety of tests have been used to categorize these patients, including MRI and cerebrospinal fluid analysis. However, the definitive diagnosis is often not made until the postmortem.[14]

Therapy
A combination of immunosuppressive drugs and corticosteroids has been used to treat MUO and the improvement in short-term survival from this type of therapy is suggestive evidence of an autoimmune cause.[14]

Dermatologic Autoimmune Diseases
The skin is an organ that is associated with a multitude of immune-mediated diseases; both allergic and autoimmune conditions affect the skin. Among the autoimmune skin diseases that afflict dogs and cats the pemphigus complex of vesicular skin diseases is of particular interest. Pemphigus is a disease that manifests as blisters (bullae) on the skin and/or mucous membranes. Although blisters are the primary lesion, patients often present with erosions that occur after the blister has been opened up by self-trauma. The complex of pemphigus includes several disorders that are differentiated by the layers of epithelial cells that are affected. The mechanism of disease pathogenesis involves the formation of autoantibodies that are directed against desmoglein, a protein that is involved in adhesion of adjacent epithelial cells within an epidermis. There are 2 types of desmoglein that are targets of the autoantibodies: desmoglein 1 and 3. In experimental studies, the desmoglein 1 antibodies have been shown to be pathogenic.[16,17]

There are at least 4 variants of pemphigus in dogs; these are pemphigus vulgaris, pemphigus foliaceus, pemphigus erythematosus, and pemphigus vegetans. The most severe form is pemphigus vulgaris, in which the lesions are deep in the epidermis, whereas in the milder form, pemphigus foliaceus, only the uppermost layers of the epidermis are affected.[3]

Pemphigus vulgaris
Description and pathogenesis Pemphigus vulgaris, the most severe of the pemphigus diseases, is recognized in dogs and cats. Formation of bullae deep in the epidermis occurs after binding of the antidesmoglein antibodies at the junction of the cells. These bullae ultimately rupture and result in deep and severe erosions. Pemphigus vulgaris presents with open erosive lesions on oral mucous membranes in about 90% of observed canine cases (**Fig. 3**). Systemic clinical signs often accompany the skin/mucous membrane lesions. These signs include anorexia, depression, and fever. In cats, lesions are usually associated with lips, hard palate, nasal philtrum, and gums and appear as erosions. The pathogenesis of vesicle development involves the binding

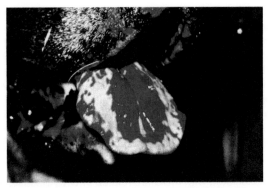

Fig. 3. Severe ulceration of the oral mucosa in a canine patient with pemphigus vulgaris.

of IgG antibodies to the desmoglein antigens that are associated with the glycocalyx of the keratinocytes with subsequent complement fixation.

Diagnosis Diagnosis of these blistering diseases is made using a combination of clinical signs and histopathology.[16,18] The use of immunofluorescence testing to localize antibody and/or complement deposition in the skin can provide additional conformational data. In pemphigus vulgaris, the location of the vesicles in the epidermis is deep, bordering on the basement membrane, creating deep erosions (**Fig. 4A**). Immunofluorescence staining with IgG reveals a honeycomb appearance that shows the presence of intercellular IgG deposition (**Fig. 4B**).

Therapy Treatment of pemphigus vulgaris and the other varieties of pemphigus involves immunosuppression, usually with prednisone and often with one of several immunosuppressive drugs (cyclosporine, chlorambucil, azathioprine). Because pemphigus vulgaris is often associated with systemic effects, supportive care is important and, because secondary infection of the lesions is likely, vigorous antibiotic therapy must be included in the treatment plan. The prognosis is generally poor.

Pemphigus foliaceus
Description and pathogenesis This condition is the most common form of pemphigus in both dogs and cats. It is characterized by hair loss, scabs, and sometimes erosions

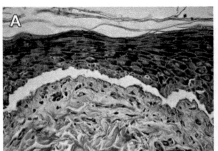
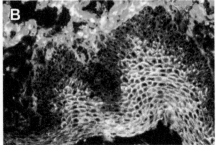

Fig. 4. (A) Histology showing cleft formed from immune attack on epidermis (hematoxylin-eosin, original magnification ×200). (B) Immunofluorescent staining of a tissue sample from a patient with pemphigus shows the binding of IgG in a honeycomb pattern showing the antibody recognition of the desmoglein protein between adjacent epithelial cells in the epidermis. Frozen section stained with fluorescein isothiocyanate conjugated anti-canine IgG (original magnification ×200).

on the ears and face (**Fig. 5**). The pathogenesis is similar to that described for pemphigus vulgaris but the location of the lesions is more superficial in the epidermis.

Diagnosis Suggestive clinical signs and skin biopsy for histology and immunofluorescence are used to obtain the diagnosis.

Therapy Immunosuppressive drugs are generally effective and in some cases can be discontinued after recovery.

Bullous pemphigoid

Description and pathogenesis Bullous pemphigoid is another variant of the autoimmune blistering diseases. It is the second most common of this disease category in dogs and cats.[18] The autoantibodies are directed against collagen XVII epitopes and lesions are generally located on nonmucosal skin.[19] There is an uncommon variant referred to as mucus membrane (cicatricial) pemphigoid. In this disease there are autoantibodies directed against basement membrane proteins.[19]

Diagnosis Histopathology of the skin biopsy in patients with suggestive lesions shows subepidermal vesicles containing neutrophils and eosinophils.[18]

Therapy

Treatment with tetracycline and niacinamide is used initially with the addition of a glucocorticoid if needed. Prognosis is good.

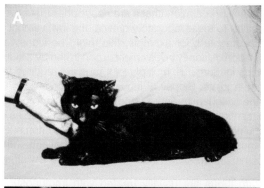

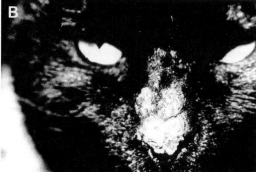

Fig. 5. (*A*) Typical appearance of a cat with pemphigus foliaceus. (*B*) The cat's ears have dry crusty lesions.

Systemic Autoimmune Disease

Systemic lupus erythematosus

Unlike the previously discussed autoimmune diseases that are organ specific, SLE is a multisystem disease.

Description and pathogenesis Dogs and cats with SLE can present with clinical signs related to many different body systems. A common presentation is lameness (shifting leg lameness) with swollen joints, but patients can also present with kidney failure, skin lesions, or hemolytic anemia. Patients with lupus have antinuclear antibodies (ANA) present in the circulation. These ANAs bind to nuclear antigens (eg, double-stranded DNA, histones) and form immune complexes that deposit in small blood vessels, creating vasculitis because of complement fixation and attraction of neutrophils; this is characteristic of a type 3 hypersensitivity reaction.[20] Kidney glomeruli are particularly vulnerable to deposition of these immune complexes and, as the disease progresses, glomerular destruction occurs with resulting leakage of protein into the urine. The joints are most commonly affected by immune complex deposition with complement activation and the attraction of neutrophils into the synovial fluid. A joint tap on a patient with lupus reveals high numbers of neutrophils in a sterile environment. Patients with lupus that also have anemia and/or thrombocytopenia have antibodies reactive with erythrocytes and megakaryocytes.[4]

As with many autoimmune diseases, there seems to be a genetic risk associated with development of SLE. One study of Nova Scotia duck tolling retrievers identified 5 loci associated with SLE-related disease.[21]

Diagnosis The diagnosis of SLE involves several criteria: a positive ANA test or a positive lupus erythematosus cell preparation (these are neutrophils that have engulfed opsonized nuclei).[22] In addition to these laboratory criteria, the involvement of at least 2 body systems must be documented; for example, this might be kidney and skin, or joints and kidney. Determination of kidney involvement is confirmed by a kidney biopsy stained for antibody deposition in glomeruli; multiple joint taps are required to confirm immune complex involvement in joints. Biopsy of lupus-related skin lesions reveals deposition of IgG and/or C3 at the basal lamina (lupus band) when stained with immunofluorescence (**Fig. 6**). In human patients, a butterfly rash is commonly described as erythema beneath the eyes and over the nose. In dogs, lesions on the face are often seen as well, particularly on the nasal planum (**Fig. 7**). On the chemistry panel, patients with lupus often show evidence of a polyclonal gammopathy, with a corresponding low albumin/globulin ratio.

Therapy Patients with lupus are usually treated with immunosuppressive therapy: prednisone alone or in conjunction with Imuran. Often patients can be weaned off these drugs or at least onto a low dose of prednisone for maintenance. A useful way to monitor the response to therapy is to perform ANA titers monthly; a decrease in titer indicates effective therapy.

SUMMARY

There are many more autoimmune diseases that are recognized in domestic animals. The descriptions of diseases presented here provide examples to show the magnitude of immune targets and the variable nature of autoimmune diseases. Other will describe autoimmune diseases that are recognized in dogs, cats, and horses include immune-mediated thrombocytopenia, VKH (Vogt-Koyanagi-Harada) ocular disease (dogs), and Evans syndrome (which includes concurrent both immune-mediated anemia and immune-mediated thrombocytopenia).

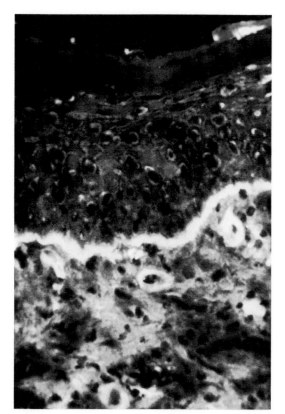

Fig. 6. A biopsy taken from the skin on the nasal planum of a dog with SLE; staining of the tissue for immunofluorescence visualization of IgG and complement binding shows a band at the dermal-epidermal junction that is referred to as a lupus band. Frozen section stained with fluorescein isothiocyanate conjugated anti-canine IgG (original magnification ×400).

Newly Recognized Autoimmune Diseases

There are several inflammatory diseases that seem to have a genetic association with 1 or more purebred dog breeds (eg, sebaceous adenitis) and researchers are attempting to determine whether these conditions are emerging autoimmune

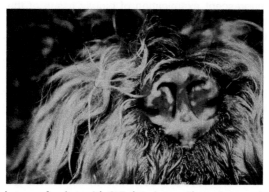

Fig. 7. The nasal planum of a dog with SLE showing erythematous and erosive lesions.

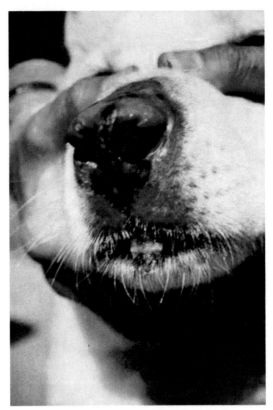

Fig. 8. This dog was diagnosed with discoid lupus. ANA negative and only the skin was affected. These lesions are often exacerbated by exposure to sunlight.

diseases.[23] Veterinary immunologists often look to the human example for documentation of possible immune-mediated diseases that might occur in their patients, and they frequently are able to find them. One such case is the newly described autoimmune skin disease called generalized discoid lupus erythematosus (GDLE). Banovic and colleagues[24] studied 10 dogs that met the criteria for this condition as described for humans. The presence of lesions that show a characteristic lupus band on immunofluorescent examination of biopsy tissue of the nasal planum is common in dogs with sun exposure and is referred to as discoid lupus (**Fig. 8**). These patients are ANA negative, do not have systemic signs, and the lesions are limited to the face. In contrast, the dogs diagnosed with GDLE had low ANA titers and a lupus band with deposition of IgG and/or IgM and/or C3 at the dermoepidermal junction. Several treatments were tried, including glucocorticoids with cyclosporine with ketoconazole, or topical tacrolimus 0.1% ointment and oral hydroxychloroquine, or a tetracycline/niacinamide combination. Full details of these cases have been reported.[24]

REFERENCES

1. Mackay IR. Travels and travails of autoimmunity: a historical journey from discovery to rediscovery. Autoimmun Rev 2010;9(5):A251–8.

2. Murphy K, Weaver C. Janeway's immunobiology. 9th edition. Garland Science; 2017.

3. Tizard IR. Veterinary immunology. 10th edition. Elsevier; 2012.

4. Gershwin LJ. Case studies in veterinary immunology. Garland Science; 2017.

5. Whitley NT, Day MJ. Immunomodulatory drugs and their application to the management of canine immune-mediated disease. J Small Anim Pract 2011;52(2): 70–85.

6. McLachlan SM, Rapoport B. Breaking tolerance to thyroid antigens: changing concepts in thyroid autoimmunity. Endocr Rev 2014;35(1):59–105.

7. Nelson RW, Reusch CE. Animal models of disease: classification and etiology of diabetes in dogs and cats. J Endocrinol 2014;222(3):T1–9.

8. Boag AM, Christie MR, McLaughlin KA, et al. Autoantibodies against Cytochrome P450 side-chain cleavage enzyme in dogs (Canis lupus familiaris) affected with hypoadrenocorticism (Addison's disease). PLoS One 2015; 10(11):e0143458.

9. Cartwright JA, Stone J, Rick M, et al. Polyglandular endocrinopathy type II (Schmidt's syndrome) in a Dobermann pinscher. J Small Anim Pract 2016; 57(9):491–4.

10. Kooistra HS, Rijnberk A, van den Ingh TS. Polyglandular deficiency syndrome in a boxer dog: thyroid hormone and glucocorticoid deficiency. Vet Q 1995;17(2): 59–63.

11. Dewey CW, Bailey CS, Shelton GD, et al. Clinical forms of acquired myasthenia gravis in dogs: 25 cases (1988-1995). J Vet Intern Med 1997;11(2):50–7.

12. Hague DW, Humphries HD, Mitchell MA, et al. Risk factors and outcomes in cats with acquired myasthenia gravis (2001-2012). J Vet Intern Med 2015;29(5): 1307–12.

13. Wolf Z, Vernau K, Safra N, et al. Association of early onset myasthenia gravis in Newfoundland dogs with the canine major histocompatibility complex class I. Neuromuscul Disord 2017;27(5):409–16.

14. Cornelis I, Volk HA, Van Ham L, et al. Prognostic factors for 1-week survival in dogs diagnosed with meningoencephalitis of unknown aetiology. Vet J 2016; 214:91–5.

15. Schrauwen I, Barber RM, Schatzberg SJ, et al. Identification of novel genetic risk loci in Maltese dogs with necrotizing meningoencephalitis and evidence of a shared genetic risk across toy dog breeds. PLoS One 2014;9(11):e112755.

16. Blair RV, Wakamatsu N, Pucheu-Haston CM. Pathology in practice. Pemphigus vulgaris. J Am Vet Med Assoc 2015;246(4):419–21.

17. Bizikova P, Dean GA, Hashimoto T, et al. Cloning and establishment of canine desmocollin-1 as a major autoantigen in canine pemphigus foliaceus. Vet Immunol Immunopathol 2012;149(3–4):197–207.

18. Olivry T, Linder KE. Dermatoses affecting desmosomes in animals: a mechanistic view of acantholytic blistering skin diseases. Vet Dermatol 2009;20(5–6):313–26.

19. Olivry T, Jackson HA. Diagnosing new autoimmune blistering skin diseases of dogs and cats. Clin Tech Small Anim Pract 2001;16(4):225–9.

20. Gershwin LJ. Antinuclear antibodies in domestic animals. Ann N Y Acad Sci 2005;1050:364–70.

21. Bannasch D, Andersson G, Hansson-Hamlin H, et al. Genome-wide association mapping identifies multiple loci for a canine SLE-related disease complex. Nat Genet 2010;42(3):250–4.

22. Jones DR. Canine systemic lupus erythematosus: new insights and their implications. J Comp Pathol 1993;108(3):215–28.

23. Pedersen NC, Brucker L, Tessier NG, et al. The effect of genetic bottlenecks and inbreeding on the incidence of two major autoimmune diseases in standard poodles, sebaceous adenitis and Addison's disease. Canine Genet Epidemiol 2015; 2:14.
24. Banovic F, Linder KE, Uri M, et al. Clinical and microscopic features of generalized discoid lupus erythematosus in dogs (10 cases). Vet Dermatol 2016;27(6): 488-e131.

Printed and bound by CPI Group (UK) Ltd, Croydon, CR0 4YY

07/10/2024

01040502-0013